T0248852

Advances and Issues in Kidney Transplantation

Advances and Issues in Kidney Transplantation

Edited by **Reagen Hu**

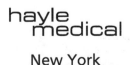

New York

Published by Hayle Medical,
30 West, 37th Street, Suite 612,
New York, NY 10018, USA
www.haylemedical.com

Advances and Issues in Kidney Transplantation
Edited by Reagen Hu

© 2015 Hayle Medical

International Standard Book Number: 978-1-63241-024-5 (Hardback)

This book contains information obtained from authentic and highly regarded sources. Copy-right for all individual chapters remain with the respective authors as indicated. A wide variety of references are listed. Permission and sources are indicated; for detailed attributions, please refer to the permissions page. Reasonable efforts have been made to publish reliable data and information, but the authors, editors and publisher cannot assume any responsibility for the validity of all materials or the consequences of their use.

The publisher's policy is to use permanent paper from mills that operate a sustainable forestry policy. Furthermore, the publisher ensures that the text paper and cover boards used have met acceptable environmental accreditation standards.

Trademark Notice: Registered trademark of products or corporate names are used only for explanation and identification without intent to infringe.

Printed in the United States of America.

Contents

Preface

This book highlights important areas of scientific research in kidney transplantation. It discusses the most novel methodologies in transplantation immunology. Aspects of daily care of transplant recipients are also elucidated in this all-inclusive book. The aim of this book is to enhance the care instruments for all the patients and serve as a useful source of reference.

Significant researches are present in this book. Intensive efforts have been employed by authors to make this book an outstanding discourse. This book contains the enlightening chapters which have been written on the basis of significant researches done by the experts.

Finally, I would also like to thank all the members involved in this book for being a team and meeting all the deadlines for the submission of their respective works. I would also like to thank my friends and family for being supportive in my efforts.

Editor

Clinical Aspects of Renal Transplantation

Kidney Transplantation Techniques

Farzad Kakaei, Saman Nikeghbalian and
Seyed Ali Malekhosseini

Additional information is available at the end of the chapter

1. Introduction

First successful kidney transplantation was done over 60 years ago and now because of major advances in immunosuppressive medicine, this represents the treatment of choice for patients with end-stage renal disease (ESRD). The kidney was the first organ to be transplanted regularly, and it remains the most common organ transplanted today but the surgical technique has changed very little from the original pelvic operation during this long period.

In most cases kidney is placed retroperitoneally and the iliac arteries and veins are used for perfusion of this organ and the ureter is transplanted directly to the bladder. But the sophisticated intensive care units and advanced perioperative anesthetic techniques lead to the use of more marginal donors for more complicated recipients. Now using a kidney graft from a donor after cardiac death or proceeding to kidney transplantation as a part of multivisceral or other abdominal organ transplantation is a routine procedure in the major transplant centers of the world. In such conditions the kidney grafts are not harvested in an optimized preoperative planning and may be damaged during the surgery. Then we may confront with a graft with 2 or more delicate or very short arteries or veins, ruptured capsule or transected ureter. We may use grafts with congenital anomalies such as horseshoe kidneys or duplicated ureteral system. Also the recipient procedure may be her or his second, third or more transplantation surgery and no more iliac vessels remained for anastomosis and the bladder may be so damaged that makes the anastomosis of the ureter to the bladder impossible. The transplant surgeon should always be ready to conquer such challenges. Using an intraperitoneal space, using the aorta or inferior vena cava or other major arteries and veins such as splenic vessels, and the native ureters for reconstruction of the urine outflow should be an in-hand procedure for every transplant surgeon.

In this chapter we will review basic steps of the standard approach to recipient's procedure from preparing the graft, then the skin incision till the skin closure with special attention to basic vascular and urinary tract re-establishment techniques and also intraoperative care of the patient. Then we proceed to the special and unusual situations including: complex vascular and ureteral reconstruction techniques, using kidneys with congenital and other anatomical anomalies, en bloc double kidney transplantation, using other vasculature for transplanting the kidney in different intraperitoneal spaces, and kidney transplantation conjoint with other abdominal organs.

2. Graft preparation

Preservation of the viability of the graft during the time between explantation and implantation is vital for early and late graft function after transplantation. Most kidney transplant teams consist of at least two separate groups. One group prepares the donor and the other team is doing the recipient operation at the same time or with some delay depending on the duration needs for transferring the graft from the donor operating room to the recipient operation theatre. In many countries such as the United States or in the Euro Zone the kidney grafts from the deceased donors are transferred between hospitals, cities or even countries according to the Human Leukocyte Antigen (HLA) matching or other important criteria for attributing the graft to a preferred recipient. In such conditions it's better to use every effort to improve the graft longevity. Using better preservation solutions or automatic machine perfusion systems are among the routine measurements in such conditions which are discussed in other chapters of this book. The surgeons and coordinators should shorten the ischemic time of the graft as long as possible and during all of this period the temperature of the graft should be maintained between 1-4° centigrade to decrease the injury to the graft.

Simple hypothermia is not enough for preserving the viability of the graft and evacuation of the graft blood and replacing it with a preservation solution is a mandatory step in the graft preparation. Graft cold irrigation in the deceased donors is done during the harvesting operation by irrigation of the clamped aorta and the solution used for this irrigation may be any of the pre-prepared solutions such as Belzer University of Wisconsin's (UW), Histidine-Tryptophan-Ke-toglutarate (HTK, Bretschneider or Custodiol), Euro-Collins, Celsior or other newer solutions such as Biolasol® (Dolińska B, et al, 2012)[1]. Table 1 shows the compositions of some of these solutions. All of the blood should be evacuated from the graft during this phase. In the living donor, all of the irrigation is done after removing the graft the donor body in an iced cold basin. In the countries that the living donor still forms over 75% of the donor pool such as China or India, irrigation of the living donor graft is done by more simple solutions such as lactated Ringer's solution and many studies shows that when the total ischemic time is less than 60 minutes (as in most living donor programs) the long-term graft survival is not impacted significantly by using these simple solutions comparing with more complex solutions (Prasad GS, et al, 2007)[2]. In our center we add lidocaine (100 mg/liter), sodium bicarbonate (10 meq/liter) and heparin (5000 IU/liter) to this simple solution. Also, we use intravenous Mannitol and Furosemide in the donor just before the arterial clamping for better diuresis before nephrectomy.

Name	Composition	Claimed advantages
Belzer UW solution (Viaspan®)	Potassium lactobionate: 100 mmol/l KH_2PO_4: 25 mmol/l $MgSO_4$: 5 mmol/l Raffinose: 30 mmol/l Adenosine: 5 mmol/l Glutathione: 3 mmol/l Allopurinol: 1 mmol/l Hydroxyethyl starch: 50 g/l	Allows for kidney preservation time up to 48 hours Allows for liver preservation time up to 24 hours Allows for pancreas preservation time up to 24 hours Provides enough time to admit patients from distant locations Provides enough time to improve recipient matching Provides enough time to operate in a semi-elective situation
Histidine-Tryptophan-Ketoglutarate (Custodiol®)	Sodium chloride: 15 mmol/l Potassium chloride: 9 mmol/l Potassium hydrogen 2-Ketoglutarate: 1mmol/l Magnesium chloride: 4 mmol/l Histidine · HCl:18.0 mmol/l Histidine: 180 mmol/l Tryptophan: 2 mmol/l Mannitol: 30 mmol/l Calcium chloride: 0.015 mmol/l	Rapid homogenous cooling due to low viscosity Superior recovery of function Excellent ischemic tolerance Virtual absence of side effects Simple perfusion technique (ready-to-use, no additives or preparation)
Celsior	Mannitol 60 mmol/l Lactobionic Acid 80 mmol/l Glutamtic Acid 20 mmol/l Histidine 30 mmol/l Calcium Chloride 0.25 mmol/l Potassium Chloride 15 mmol/l Magnesium Chloride 13 mmol/l Sodium Hydroxide 100 mmol/l Reduced Glutathione 3 mmol/l	low potassium comparing with UW prevention of tissue edema prevention of free radical damage prevention of calcium overload with adequate buffer Better for heart and lung transplantation (as depicted by its manufacturer, Genzyme)
Euro-Collins (Renograf®)	Potassium phosphate 42.5 mmol.l Potassium chloride 15 mmol/l Sodium bicarbonate 10 mmol/l Anhydrous glucose 35 g/l Mannitol 31.7 mmol/l Raffinose 3.5 mmol/l	Preserves the kidney up to 48 hours An out of date solution in most US and European centers

Table 1. Composition of the more common organ preservation solutions.

When possible, the donor team should report the detailed graft anatomy (including number of arteries, veins and ureters and any anatomical anomaly or inadvertent injury to the graft during the donor operation) to the recipient team, especially when the graft is transferred from another hospital locally or regionally. It is very important to prevent any more injury to the graft and its capsule, vessels or ureter during the back table procedure, especially in case of deceased donor grafts which usually accompanied with other abdominal organs or at least covered by the peritoneum or peri-renal fats or other non-important tissues. Direct contact of the ice with the graft should be prevented by inserting the graft in a separate basin or organ bag filled with a cold solution and then inserting this bag in another iced filled basin.

First of all, for irrigation of the living donor graft, the surgeon should find the artery and canulate it with an atraumatic olive-headed heparin irrigation needle as shown in figure 1. Using other devices such as Angiocath©, Baranule© or any types of intravenous needles for irrigation should be discouraged because of risk of intimal injury induced by such cannulas. In many cases, it may be difficult to find the artery first because it is hidden by other hilar tissues or retracted to the deeper hilar areas of the graft. In such conditions the irrigation may be started by canulation the more accessible renal vein, till the surgeon finds the artery. All the dissections should better be done after complete irrigation. At this point all of the renal parenchyma will appear in yellow-pink color. All of the dissections should be done delicately by using atraumatic or microvascular instruments, without any more injury to the vessels intima or their major branches and any more unusual traction of the vessel wall.

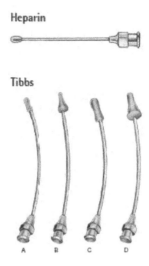

Figure 1. Special olive-headed needles for irrigation (Courtesy of GEISTER Medizintechnik GmbH, Tuttlingen/ Germany)

When using the left kidney of the living donor the adrenal and gonadal vein should be on the graft in order to have a longer vein for future anastomosis. In both right or left kidneys or living donor or deceased donor grafts, the surgeon should make every effort to preserve the connective tissues between the ureter and the gonadal vein to prevent ischemic injury to the delicate collateral vessels of the ureter. Always the ureter should be accompanied by at least one centimeter of the peri-ureteral tissues and also the hilar inferior triangle (e.g. the window between the inferior pole of the graft and the ureteral origin from the renal pelvis) should be maintained intact. Removing peri-renal fat or other tissues should be postponed till complete renal revascularization. These tissues are protective for handling of the graft and might be used for graft covering or anchoring during or after revascularization.

The window between the renal artery and vein in the renal hilum is full of accessory branches and lymphatic vessel. All of the major arterial branches especially of the inferior pole should be maintained intact. Any injury to this branches leads to regional ischemia or necrosis of the kidney or ureter which may lead to future graft dysfunction or ischemia – induced hypertension in the donor or ureteral necrosis, ureteral anastomosis disruption or urine leakage. Some surgeons suggest that all of the major lymphatic vessels should be ligated to prevent future lymphocele, however, the most important measurement for preventing the lymphocele is avoiding excessive dissections around the iliac artery during the preparing the implantation site.

The best approach for prevention of arterial branch injury is to start with dissection of the renal vein and follow its wall through the hilum until sufficient length is achieved by ligating the minor veins. We suture-ligate the accessory minor vein branches and also the major lumbar veins by 6-0 Prolene suture for prevention of postoperative bleeding from hilar vessels.

If the graft has more than one artery, vein or ureter, the surgeon should decide which type of reconstruction is suitable according to the condition of the graft and the recipient. In the deceased donor it's better to use a Carrel patch of aorta and inferior vena cava in line with the graft vessels. But this has two major impacts on future graft implantation. First, this results in a longer than usual artery (especially in the right side) or vein (especially in the left side) which may be results in kinking (and future thrombosis or hypertension) after the anastomosis. And second, it will results in a large Carrel patch in some cases. The surgeon has to remove a large patch from the recipient's vessels for a good anastomosis. If complicated by graft non-function, then future removal of the graft will result in a large defect of the recipient vessels which will be dangerous or even limb life threatening. Also, the Carrel patch of the aorta may be severely atherosclerotic and could not be used for a safe anastomosis. Any reconstruction will elongate the total ischemic time of the graft, and we should do every effort to prevent this by postponing unnecessary dissections and reconstructions to the time after at least partial reperfusion of the graft.

According to these important issues, when possible, we prefer to use no reconstruction prior to implantation to decrease the ischemic time. Every transplant surgeon should be fully trained and familiar with microvascular techniques in such conditions. Every arterial branch should be anastomosed separately. The major artery is anastomosed first usually to the internal iliac artery, which provides a longer arterial conduit and allow more free movements of the graft for venous anastomosis. Smaller arteries are anastomosed after reperfusion of the graft to the external iliac artery or even to the smaller arteries such as inferior epigastric artery (El-Sherbiny M, et al, 2008)[3]. When all arterial branches have the same size, then reperfusion is postponed till the end of anastomosis of all of the arterial branches usually to the external iliac artery but if the kidney has a large artery and some other smaller arteries then reperfusion is started after completion of the large artery anastomosis. Arteries less than 1 mm could be ligated specially in the upper pole. Also ligation of the arteries with resultant ischemic area of less than 15% of the upper or middle pole is acceptable and by reducing the total operation duration will reduce the complications in the recipient comparing with adding a long microvascular anastomosis to the operation. Arteries larger than 1 mm in the lower pole should be reperfused by anastomosis if possible to prevent ischemia of the ureter.

If the surgeon decides to reconstruct the arteries before implantation then multiple varieties of techniques could be used: side to side anastomosis of the same size arteries or end to side anastomosis of a small artery to a larger artery. Using microvascular techniques with a good illumination and at least 4.5X magnification and 7-0 or 8-0 Prolene sutures, all of the ties should be placed out of the intimal surface and the lumen should be protected by a smooth metal probe to prevent inadvertent back-wall suturing. In the deceased donor, the surgeon can use freely every small bifurcated or trifurcated donor artery (such as the celiac artery) for these delicate reconstructions. In such complex situations such as severe atherosclerosis of the renal artery orifice when eversion endarterectomy is not possible (Nghiem DD, Choi SS, 1992) [4] or results in a damaged artery, the best approach for salvage of the graft is transecting the diseased part of the renal artery and using a small branch of the donor artery such as the left gastric or splenic artery as an elongation conduit of the renal artery. In the case of living donors, a short segment of the recipient saphenous vein may be a good choice for this purpose but it has a real risk of future aneurismal transformation in the future (Sharma A, et al, 2010) [5]. Sometimes we could use a combination of these techniques. For example when the graft has 2 large-size and 1 small-size artery, the best option is to perform an anastomosis between the small-size artery and one of the larger size branches and then perform two separate anastomoses in the recipient. This action will reduce the total operative time of the recipient.

Approach to the vein branches is a little different because of intra-parenchymal communications between the vein branches. We could ligate non-major venous branches, but when the vein branches are in the same size we should reconstruct them before venous anastomosis. Some surgeons prefer to mobilize the external iliac vein by ligating the internal iliac vein or superior gluteal vein or other side branches of this vein, but usually these maneuvers are futile in providing better window for venous anastomosis especially when we use the right kidney from a living donor. In such conditions we prefer to perform the venous anastomosis first or placing the graft in an upside down direction (ureter in the upper part) (Webb J et al, 2003) [6]. In the deceased donor, using a part of the donor external iliac, internal jugular or inferior vena cava as an extension graft is more preferable for adding the length of the vein graft. Such reconstructions should be done in the back table prior to implantation.

In our opinion, ureteral reconstruction also should be discouraged in case of multiple graft ureters. When the ureters have insufficient length, or denuded in their entire length, mobilization of the recipient bladder or using of the recipient ureter is preferred.

At the end of graft preparation some authors suggest that the graft should be wrapped in iced or cold saline soaked surgical gauzes or cloth stockinet or surgical glove to remain cold throughout the implantation procedure. In our opinion this is a time consuming and fruitless maneuver when the surgeons could do the anastomoses rapidly. Also using the ice packets in the site of implantation is not necessary.

3. Implantation site

So many factors impact the surgeon's decision on which site he could implant the kidney graft (table 2). These factors include: the graft size comparing with the recipient, the size, length and number of graft arteries, veins and/or ureters, previous surgeries (for example previous failed kidney transplantation, previous pelvic exploration for bladder reconstruction or anti-reflux surgeries), associated abdominal organ (liver, pancreas or small bowel) transplantation, laterality of the donor kidney (left or right), anomalies of the donor graft (horseshoe kidney, double pelvis, double ureter, etc.), and at last the number of kidney grafts (double kidney from a pediatric or old age or marginal donor). Traditionally the right iliac fossa is the standard fossa for a kidney transplantation procedure and the left iliac fossa is the preferred site for simultaneous kidney-pancreas transplantation. In the pediatric recipient when the graft is larger than usual we should use the main abdominal fossa for implantation. The most important limiting factor for each of these procedures is the length of the renal vein and also the length of the donor ureter and mobility of the recipient urinary bladder. In most instances when the recipient internal iliac artery is used as the arterial inflow, it provides a good length for mobilization and would not be a limiting factor. The right iliac fossa is the preferred site because of the more superficial position of the external iliac vein. The deep branches of the iliac vein can be suture ligated and cut if more superficialization is needed. If the recipient ureter is not diseased it can be used for urinary outflow reconstruction if the donor ureter is short.

Factor	Preferred Site	Rationale
Graft size comparing with the recipient	Abdominal fossa if the graft is very large	Prevention of kidney compartment syndrome
The size, length and number of graft arteries and veins	Iliac fossa is preferred	Prevention of entering to the abdominal cavity and postoperative ileus
The size, length and number of ureters	Iliac fossa is preferred if the recipient ureter is not diseased. Retrovesical area if the ureters are short but vessels are long enough	Prevention of urine leakage or ureteral stricture
Previous surgeries	Opposite iliac fossa	Prevention of vessel or visceral injury, prevention of lymphocele, shorter operative time
Associated abdominal organ transplantation	Left iliac fossa and in the retroperitoneal space Abdominal cavity for en bloc or composite grafts	Prevention of adding the complications of each graft on the other graft
Laterality of the donor kidney (left or right)	It's better to use right iliac fossa	More superficial position of iliac vein Some authors use the opposite side because of position of the transplanted graft for future percutaneous interventions on the urinary system
The number of kidney grafts	Retroperitoneal space of right iliac fossa	If the iliac arteries are not large enough it's better to use the abdominal aorta and inferior vena cava
Anomalies of the donor graft	Abdominal cavity if the graft is large, if the graft is small iliac fossa is better.	Enough space for the graft and enough stations for vascular anastomosis

Table 2. Factors influencing the choice of implantation site

4. Skin preparation and incision

Skin preparation and drape is not so different from other clean abdominal operations. The patient should bathe before entering the operation theatre. Hair removal is better done with hair clippers immediately before surgery. We use scrub povidone iodine or any types of alcoholic or polyethylene glycol type solutions (e.g. Decocept®) for initial washing and then normal povidone iodine for 2 times for the final preparation. Also we use a sterile (Opsite®) drape for complete covering of the incision region. The standard skin incision is the traditional hockey-stick Gibson incision or an oblique Rutherford Morison in the right iliac fossa. Gibson incision starts at the tubercule of pubis and continued laterally transverse to inguinal ligament and then upward in a curvilinear manner in the lateral border of the rectus abdominis muscle till 1-2 cm above the level of umbilicus. In larger adults extension till the anterior superior iliac spine may be enough. The epigastric vessels and the round ligament in females usually need to be ligated and transected, but the spermatic cord simply retracted medially by releasing the border of inguinal canal. The surgeon should avoid entering the peritoneal space and any defect in the peritoneum should be repaired before continuing the incision.

All the dissections should be accompanied by strict hemostasis and avoiding extreme injury to the abdominal wall muscles to simplify the future abdominal wall repair at the end of the procedure. All the bleeding sites should be completely hemostatized during this time because at the end of the procedure hemostasis will be very difficult. Also most renal failure patients has bleeding tendency due to platelet dysfunction specially in the first 2 hours after the hemodialysis or in those patient who underwent preemptive renal transplantation. If hemostasis is not complete wound or peri-graft hematoma is inevitable which will lead to the other complications such as infection, dehiscence, hydronephrosis or kidney compartment syndrome due to compression to the graft.

After entering the retroperitoneal space and revealing the anatomy of the iliac vessels and their suitability for transplantation, the iliac vein should be prepared first by ligating all lymphatics around it. It's better to avoid the first major deep iliac lymph node (Cloquet's node). Dissections around the external iliac artery should be limited and if the internal iliac artery has a good contour and length, it's better to use it as the arterial inflow. If this artery has atherosclerotic plaques an endarterectomy could be done. We use the external iliac artery only when the internal iliac artery of the other side is used previously, or when a large size discrepancy is revealed or severe atherosclerosis reduce the arterial flow to a very low and crucial level. Using the internal iliac artery slightly increases the postoperative lymphocele because of more dissections needed for its releasing, but if the surgeon ligate all the lymphatics it would not be a major problem.

Without a good exposure, transplantation is a very difficult procedure and using a, Denis-Browne (Figure 2), Kirschner(Figure 3) or Bookwalter-type (Figure 4) self retaining retractor is a critical step in the implantation procedure. Many manufacturers have invented more powerful retractors. Some of them like Thompson® retractor, although are very useful and unique for liver or kidney-pancreas transplantation, but their use for kidney transplantation alone is time consuming and is best limited to super-obese recipients. Some of them such as Henley or Darling or Gosset abdominal retractor only are useful in pediatric or thin patients with a shallow pelvis. Balfour and Balfour-Baby, Collin and Baby Collin, Ricard and Sullivan- O'Connor have the same problem. Some of them such as Omni-Flex® (Omni-Tract® surgical, Minnesota Scientific, MN, USA) or SynFrame® retractor systems (Synthes® Spine Inc., PA, USA) are modifications to the original Thompson retractor but their use may be more sophisticated.

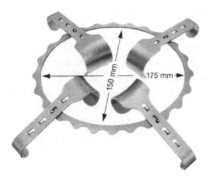

Figure 2. Denis-Browne retractor

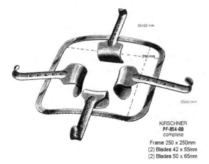

Figure 3. Kirschner retractor

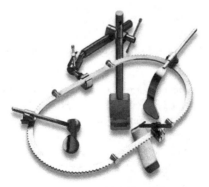

Figure 4. Bookwalter retractor

5. Vascular anastomosis

After preparation of the place of the implantation, the surgeon should transfer the graft to its position transiently for better evaluation of the anastomoses sites. Some authors suggest that slush ice should put in the bed of the graft in the recipient, but we absolutely disagree with this opinion, because the total vascular reconstruction time is usually less than 20 minutes and adding ice only increase the risk of local hypothermic injury. The surgeon should do his best efforts to reduce the total arterial and venous clamping time. First the site of each anastomosis and the position of the graft should be specified accurately according to the size and length of the vessels and also the length of the ureter and position of the recipient bladder or ureter and the final position of the implanted kidney. As described previously, we prefer to use the internal iliac artery and external iliac vein for vascular anastomoses. For reducing the vein clamping time (with subsequent risk of deep vein thrombosis), we perform the arterial anastomosis first. But when the vein is shorter than usual or when the left iliac fossa is used for implantation, or when the abdominal cavity and aorta and inferior vena cava or the external iliac artery are used for implantation, it's better to perform the venous anastomosis first.

The principles of vascular anastomosis are not different from any standard vascular surgery. The best suture size is usually 5-0 and 6-0 Prolene® sutures for venous and arterial anastomosis. The size of the needles depends of the location of the anastomosis but in most cases the needle should be taper-point or taper-cutting-tip round-bodied 3/8 circle with 11 – 13 mm length for better performance. For smaller arteries 7-0 or 8-0, 1/2 circle, 7-9.3 mm needles may be more suitable. For severe atherosclerotic arteries use of special visible Ethicon Visi-Black® Everpoint®, or Tapercut® needles with spatulated heads which is more firm and crash-resistant is needed.

After confirming the exact length and position of the anastomosis site to prevent kinking or rotation, vascular clamps are applied to the first vessel. We prefer to use Bulldog clamps to the internal iliac artery and iliac veins and Satinsky clamps for side-clamping of external iliac and common iliac artery or aorta or inferior vena cava. We discourage systemic heparinization before clamping because of bleeding tendency in chronic renal failure patients, but other authors recommend this. Heparinized saline is enough for irrigation of the vessels during the anastomosis.

For end-to-side anastomoses a patch from the vessel should be removed for preventing future constriction. This patch is removed from the arteries by No. 3, 4 or 5 aortic punches depending on the arterial size and by special Metzenbaum or Potts scissors from the veins. Also we should avoid the venous valve site in the external iliac vein, if possible. The wall of the vein is very thin proximal to the venous valves (sinuses of Valsalva) and may be ruptured during the anastomosis.

For end-to side anastomosis of a renal artery to the external iliac or common iliac or aorta, the graft artery should be spatulated in the direction of its lower corner. For end-to-end anastomosis of the renal artery to the internal iliac artery, the renal artery should be spatulated from the upper corner and the internal iliac artery should be spatulated in the direction of the opposite lower corner (in other words in the direction the deep part of the artery). Renal vein usually needs no spatulation.

An endarterectomy should be done with extreme caution after cutting the internal iliac artery or entering the external iliac artery. No intimal flaps in the opposite direction of the blood flow should be remained at the end of endarterectomy. If such flap is remained, then the surgeon should decide to change the arterial anastomosis site, if possible, or at least the flap must completely secured to the arterial wall with a tagging U-stitch.

Special attention should be paid to the length of the right artery and left renal vein of the deceased donor. They are both too long for anastomosis and if not trimmed or shortened, kinking will be inevitable which will result in postoperative renal dysfunction and hypertension.

Arterial anastomosis is started by two corner stitch in each side of the vessel as described first by Carrel in 1902. Care is taken to include equal bites of all layers of the arterial wall in each passage of the needle and the adventitia remained outside. For this purpose we perform a 1 mm adventitiectomy of both arteries and use microvascular forceps, scissors and needle holders for arterial anastomosis and also recommend using a 4.5-6X loop for magnification and surgical headlights for better illumination. It's so important that the posterior layer suturing of the arterial anastomosis is done first and from outside. The needle should move from inside to outside of the more diseased artery (usually the recipient artery) to tag the intima to the media of the artery and preventing from creating an intimal flap which will be a good trigger point for future thrombosis. The upper suture is tied but the lower is maintained untied till the end of the anastomosis. The posterior layer is sutured first and then anterior layer anastomosis is started from both corners. In the children or for small arteries at least one half of the anastomosis should be done by separate sutures. In all other continuous anastomoses (artery or vein), we tie the last suture loosely and preserve a "Growth factor" or "expansion factor" to prevent purse-string effect of the continuous suture on constricting the anastomosis as first described by Starzl in the portal anastomosis of liver transplantation (Starzl TE, 1984, Zomorrodi, et al, 2012) [7, 8]) [7].

For vein anastomosis we use a somewhat different technique. After inserting the two corner stitches, an anchoring or stay suture is used in the midpoint of the anterior layer of the venotomy site of the external iliac vein to maintain the orifice of the anastomosis site totally exposed and prevent from inadvertent catching of the posterior suture line in the anterior suture line. All the anastomosis is performed circumferentially by a single stitch that used as the proximal corner stitch. Then the surgeon should be cautious when tying this suture that the two remaining part are in the same length. The anastomosis is started from the proximal part by entering tying the corner stitch. Then the needle is entered from the posterior layer of the internal iliac vein into its lumen. Then a four-point technique is used for approximating the two intimal layers of the renal vein and external iliac vein. After completing the posterior layer then the anastomosis is continued from distal and proximal corner to the anterior layer and the anchoring stitch is removed. Again a "Growth factor" is necessary to prevent the purse string effect and also in the pediatric group, the anterior layer stitches should be in separate manner for make future growth possible. If the venotomy site is larger than the orifice of the renal vein, then after completing the posterior layer, the excessive part should be repaired before starting the anterior layer, preferably by another suture line.

6. Unusual situations

In case of thrombosed or fibrotic external iliac vein (due to multiple previous femoral vein canulations or previous DVT) or severe atherosclerotic iliac arteries, the best approach is to use the abdominal major vasculature for renal transplantation. The surgeon may decide to use the common iliac artery or vein if spared from the disease or close the wound and explore the opposite iliac fossa if preoperative Investigations or intraoperative sonographywere negative for the same complication. In extreme cases when the IVC is also thrombosed or fibrotic, or when the infrarenal aorta also is atretic or severely atherosclerotic, using the splenic or native renal vein and artery may be an option, provided that the native ureters has a normal function and anatomy.

Another unusual case is the horseshoe kidney. Anomalous vasculature is the rule in these cases. Crossed fused or non-fused ectopic kidneys have the same problem. One option for approaching this type of anomaly is to incise the ismusth between the two conjoined kidneys and use each kidney for a separate recipient. The major problem is the resultant two grafts with so many arterial and venous branches and also short and multiple ureters. Because of shortage of donor organs most centers prefer this approach. But sometimes dividing the horseshoe kidney is so difficult and may results in damaging both kidneys. In these cases it's better to use the anomalous kidney as an individual graft and use the aorta and IVC as the arterial inflow and venous outflow of the graft. Such large size graft often could not be placed retroperitoneally and should be implanted in an intraperitoneal space. The same principle is applied to double kidney grafts from a pediatric or old age or more marginal donors such as donation after cardiac death (DCD) donors: transplanting each unit separately or using the aorta and IVC as the vascular conduits of the graft. Circumaortic or retroaortic renal veins are other problematic vascular anomalies that make the transplantation procedure more difficult. In experienced hands, these anomalies per se are not contraindication for donation even from the living donors

When a suspicious lesion is found on the kidney graft, it should be incised or excised and sent for frozen section pathologic investigation. Hemostasis could be done by sutures or argon beam coagulators, following the principles of any standard partial nephrectomy. Benign lesions should be removed completely and grafts with any non-benign pathology should be discarded. Solitary cysts are very common and if small, needs no investigation. There are many case reports in the literature about transplanting kidneys from deceased donors with adult polycystic kidney disease, without any short-term complications. These grafts should only be used when the donor kidney function is good and the recipient is fully aware of the donor disease. These cases are best suitable for sedentary recipients with a short life expectancy, provided that no other contraindication such as HLA mismatch is found.

Kidney transplantation may be accompanied by pancreas, liver (Nadim MK, et al, 2012)[9], heart (Florman S, Kim-Schluger L.,2012) [10], lung (Rana RK, et al, 2011) [11] or multiorgan transplantation. In such situations usually the more important transplantation (heart, lung, liver, pancreas or small bowel) is done first. And after stability of the recipient, kidney transplantation is performed. Even when the abdomen is entered during the first procedure, it's better to use the retroperitoneal iliac fossa for the second transplant by the same incision. This will reduce the complications associated with urine leakage. In case of simultaneous kidney –pancreas transplantation the kidney transplant is done first in the left iliac fossa and during the time of this procedure, the other team prepares the pancreas graft by ex vivo surgery for the second transplantation which is usually use the right common or external iliac artery as the inflow. The kidney transplantation combined with multivisceral transplantation is usually is an en-bloc transplantation. This means that the kidney is not separated from the donor aorta and inferior vena cava (IVC). All major vascular anastomoses are done by aorta as the inflow artery and IVC and/or portal vein as the venous outflow. The urinary recon-struction is performed after complete reperfusion of all abdominal organs.

7. Declamping and reperfusion

After completing the vascular anastomoses, the opposite corner stay sutures remained untied until reperfusion. The recipient systolic blood pressure should be at least 120 mmHg and the central venous pressure between 10 to 14 cm H_2O. The use of vasopressors such as dopamine for increasing the blood pressure is controversial. Immunosuppressant is best infused before declamping according to the protocols of each transplant ward. Some authors suggests some over-hydration, infusing Furosemide and Mannitol and correction of acid-base imbalance according to the last arterial blood gas base deficit before declamping to prevent the so called "reperfusion syndrome". Unlike liver or small bowel transplantation, in most cases reperfu-sion syndrome will not be a problematic issue, because the kidney graft is relatively small, except when using an adult kidney for a pediatric recipient or in cases of a long implantation time with complete aortic or common or external iliac artery clamping time. In such cases the cause of "reperfusion syndrome" is transient ischemia of the lower limbs. The anesthesiologist should prepare sodium bicarbonate, calcium gluconate, and insulin with 50% Glucose before declamping for managing this complication and obtain an arterial blood gas before and after the declamping for estimating the severity of acidosis and monitor the electrocardiogram for diagnosis of hyperkalemia.

Arterial declamping is done first and after complete filling of the graft, veins are also opened. In this phase brisk bleeding is a rule, especially when we applied "growth factors" to the last ties. Most of the bleeding will be stopped spontaneously after complete dilatation of the anastomotic lines. Small bleeding sites may be covered by small parts of any hemostatic agent such as Surgicel®, N-butyl cyanoacrylate glues, Tachosil® or similar agents (Sageshima J, et al, 2011) [13]. All the other larger bleeding sites should be transligated or repaired by fine Prolene® sutures especially near the hilum, but extreme caution should be paid not to include the delicate hilar arterial branches in the sutures.

The kidney should be firm and well-perfused after 1-2 minutes and urine flow usually starts after that. If the graft is flaccid and the patient's blood pressure is good, arterial kinking is the first differential diagnosis. This usually is resolved by repositioning of the graft. Also the surgeon could transiently clamp the renal vein or the distal part of the external iliac artery. If not, thrombosis must be considered and ruled out as soon as possible.

8. Urinary reconstruction

After completing the reperfusion stage usually the urine flow is started. Sometimes, especially in case of deceased donors or when the nephrectomy has been performed with difficulty in the living donors, the urine flow will be delayed. If the color and contour of the graft look good and the arterial and venous flow is good with a well-palpable thrill in the hilum, the surgeon should proceed to urinary reconstruction.

First of all the urinary bladder should be filled with sterile normal saline serum through previously installed urinary catheter. Some surgeons add 10ml/lit povidone iodine and 80 mg/lit Gentamicin or 500 mg/lit Amikacin to the irrigation fluid for better sterility of the bladder (Salehipour M, et al, 2010) [13] but its effect is controversial. The kidney should be positioned in its final expected place to prevent the tension on the remained ureter before cutting the excess length of the ureter. It's better to use the smallest possible length of the ureter to reduce future ischemic complications. If this step is forgotten the final length of ureter may be shorter than expected and this will result in kinking of the vasculature and changing the location of the kidney from its ideal position.

The surgeon has many options for urinary reconstruction: ureteroneocystostomy, ureter-oureterostomy, pyeloureterostomy, and pyelocystostomy or even ureteroenterostomy to an ileal conduit or Koch (Manassero F, et al, 2011) [14] or pyelopyelostomy in case of or-thotopic kidney transplantation or complicated case (Wagner M, et al, 1994) [15]. The type of reconstruction depends on the position of the graft, the length, condition and number of the donor ureter(s), the condition of the recipient's bladder or bladder substi-tute (including its capacity and continence), previous operations on the recipient bladder or ureter (and its antireflux condition). The anastomosis should be done by absorbable sutures, usually polydioxanone sutures. Because of the risk of infection, use of any types of stents, such as double J stents or newer antireflux stents are controversial (Parapiboon W, et al, 2012) [16], but we use it in our center and remove it after 3 weeks. At least 4 techniques and their modifications are discussed in the literature for ureteroneocystosto-my (Kayler L, et al, 2010) [17]. Prevention of leakage, stricture and reflux is the final goal of all of these techniques. The two most common types are transvesical or Leadbetter-Po-litano (LP) technique and the extravesical or modified Lich-Gregoir (LG) technique. We use and recommend the second technique because it needs fewer dissections and use on-ly one small cystostomy incision (comparing with 2 large cystostomy incision needs for LP technique) with comparable antireflux characteristics and fewer complications. The LG technique can be performed in a very shorter time. After distending the bladder, the detrusor muscle dissected bluntly in the dome of the bladder approximately for a length of 3 cm till the mucosa bulges out. The ureter shortened to its ideal length and spatulated for a length of 2 cm in its anti-mesoureteral direction and then the bladder mucosa incised. Anastomosis is started near the heel of the spatulated ureter 2-3 mm in the opposite direction of the corner of the ureter. In this manner, the tie is placed outside and with some distance from the corner. The mucosa of the bladder is then sutured to the ureteral end with simple continuous sutures. After completing the anastomosis, an absorbable suture is used for approximating the detrusor muscle to close over the anastomosis and creating a small submucosal tunnel for its antireflux mechanism. The LP techniques and the two other extravesical techniques are better described in the literature (Kayler L, et al, 2010) [17]. In the LP technique, a large anterior cystostomy is done for visualization of the bladder interior and the ureter is transferred through another small posterior cystostomy and then through the mucosa and after anchoring the distal end to the mucosa, the bladder is closed in 2 layers with absorbable sutures. Another extravesical technique is the single or double U-stitch technique. In these techniques after opening the submucosal tunnel by creating by dissection of detrusor muscle and incising the bladder mucosa only 1 U-stitch (Shanfield, 1972) [18] at the toe or 2 U-stitch (MacKinnon et al, 1968) [19] at the toe and heel of the trimmed ureter is used for anchoring the ureter to bladder mucosa and then the detrussor muscle closed as the same manner of the LG technique.

Another extravesical technique uses two parallel incisions in the detrusor muscle, first posterior for transferring the ureter in a submucosal tunnel and the second incision for anastomosis of the ureter to the ureteral mucosa (Barry JM, 1983) [20]. In the last technique, the ureter is anastomosed to the bladder full-thickness wall without any antireflux mechanism (Starzl, et al, 1989) [21]. In our opinion, the surgeon should be familiar with all of these methods and use them as needed, but we have the most experience with the modified LG technique without any major urologic complication (Davari HR, et al, 2006) [22].

When the graft ureter is short, ischemic, or denuded, the surgeon should use the native ureters for ureteroureterostomy or pyeloureterostomy if they are completely in a healthy condition (no stricture, no infection, no dilation or no reflux) or decide to perform a pyeloneocystostomy. This should be done with extreme caution to prevent kinking or pressure on the graft vasculature or repositioning of the graft. A Boari flap or psoas hitch is often necessary in all cases.

In case of previous bladder surgery such as antireflux surgeries or cystoplasty or bladder augmentation, it's very important that the site of final urinary reconstruction is fully depicted before proceeding with vascular anastomosis, or even before proceeding with nephrectomy in the living donor. Also the blood supply of the tissues used for augmentation should be considered. Creating a submucosal flap in the augmented bladder may results in ischemia of the tissues used for augmentation and if possible it's better to use the native bladder area for ureteral anastomosis.

In case of double or multiple ureters (such as horseshoe kidneys or en bloc transplantation of two kidneys), the ureters can be anastomosed separately to the bladder, or one to the bladder and the shorter ones to the native ureter. Another option is anastomosis of the ureters to each other and then anastomosis of the conjoined ureter to the bladder. In our opinion using separate anastomoses (if possible) reduces the future complications.

9. Wound closure

Wound closure is the final step of the procedure. Closing is done by 2-layer repair of the abdominal muscles (first transverse and internal oblique as one layer and then the external oblique muscle), by a No. 0 loop Nylon suture. Using any drain before closure is controversial but if used it should be a closed suction drain such as a Jackson-Pratt drain and every effort should be used that the drain has no compression effect on the renal vasculature and the ureter. The exit site also should be assessed for bleeding. Every bleeding site should be assessed and repaired before closure to prevent postoperative hematoma. Diffuse oozing at the end of operation may be the result of platelet dysfunction or heparin overdose and should be managed accordingly by desmopressin and protamine sulfate, respectively. Excess perirenal fat should be removed, and the graft should be placed in a retroperitoneally created pouch parallel with the psoas muscle, to prevent compression of the kidney between the abdominal wall and the pelvic bones. If the kidney volume is greater than this space, or the renal vasculature or ureter is shorter than usual, then "compartment syndrome" is inevitable is the abdominal muscles repaired in the usual manner. In such situation, the renal artery inflow is good but the outflow will be disturbed because of pressure of the abdominal wall on the renal vein. Renal venous pressure increase and then the graft will be congested and the urine flow will decreased. If remained unmanaged, this will eventually lead to decreasing renal artery flow and finally to renal artery thrombosis and graft loss. If the surgeon could not reposition the graft in to the supravesical area and anchor it to the abdominal wall without vascular kinking, many other options should be tried. One option is to incise the rectus sheath after closing the muscles. Another option is to close the abdominal wall from distal and proximal and let the part which is covering the kidney remains unclosed or closed by an artificial mesh which is used for hernia repair. The last option is to let abdominal musculature remained completely opened and only covered by the skin. The resultant incisional hernia will be repaired in the future, usually 3 months after the transplantation. The best treatment of such conditions is "prevention" by matching the size of the donor and recipient and special attention to the length of the graft vasculature and ureter and also creating the pouch as the first step during the procedure.

Author details

Farzad Kakaei[1], Saman Nikeghbalian[2] and Seyed Ali Malekhosseini[2]

1 Tabriz University of Medical Sciences, Tabriz, Iran

2 Shiraz University of Medical Sciences, Shiraz, Iran

References

[1] Dolińska B, Ostróżka-Cieślik A, Caban A, Cierpka L, Ryszka F. Comparing the effect of Biolasol® and HTK solutions on maintaining proper homeostasis, indicating the kidney storage efficiency prior to transplantation. Ann Transplant. 2012 Jun 29;17(2): 74-8.

[2] Prasad GS, Ninan CN, Devasia A, Gnanaraj L, Kekre NS, Gopalakrishnan G.: Is Euro-Collins better than ringer lactate in live related donor renal transplantation? Indian J Urol. 2007 Jul;23(3):265-9.

[3] El-Sherbiny M, Abou-Elela A, Morsy A, Salah M, Foda A. The use of the inferior epigastric artery for accessory lower polar artery revascularization in live donor renal transplantation. Int Urol Nephrol. 2008;40(2):283-7.

[4] Nghiem DD, Choi SS. Eversion endarterectomy of the cadaver donor renal artery: a method to increase the use of elderly donor kidney allografts. J Urol. 1992 Mar;147(3): 653-5.

[5] Sharma A, King AL, Lee HM, Posner MP. Saphenous vein graft aneurysm after renal transplantation: a case report. Transplantation. 2010 May 15;89(9):1162-3.

[6] Webb J, Soomro N, Jaques B, Manas D, Talbot D. The upside down transplant kidney. Clin Transplant. 2003 Oct;17(5):484.

[7] Starzl TE, Iwatsuki S, Shaw BW Jr. A growth factor in fine vascular anastomoses. Surg Gynecol Obstet. 1984 Aug;159(2):164-5.

[8] Zomorrodi A, Kakei F, Farshi A, Zomorrodi S (2012) Is Placing an Expansion Space at the Anastomosing Site of the Vessel for Prevention of Pursiness, Safe? J Transplant Technol Res 2:113. doi:10.4172/2161-0991.1000113

[9] Nadim MK, Sung RS, Davis CL, Andreoni KA, Biggins SW, Danovitch GM, Feng S, Friedewald JJ, Hong JC, Kellum JA, Kim WR, Lake JR, Melton LB, Pomfret EA, Saab S, Genyk YS Simultaneous Liver-Kidney Transplantation Summit: Current State and Future Directions. Am J Transplant. 2012 Jul 23.

[10] Florman S, Kim-Schluger L. Organ transplantation update, part II: heart and kidney. Mt Sinai J Med. 2012 May-Jun;79(3):303-4.

[11] Rana RK, Ghandehari S, Falk JA, Simsir SA, Ghaly AS, Cheng W, Cohen JL, Peng A, Czer LS, Schwarz ER, Chaux GE. Successful combined heart-bilateral lung-kidney transplantation from a same donor to treat severe hypertrophic cardiomyopathy with secondary pulmonary hypertension and renal failure: case report and review of the literature. Transplant Proc. 2011 Sep;43(7):2820-6. Review.

[12] Sageshima J, Ciancio G, Uchida K, Romano A, Acun Z, Chen L, Burke GW 3rd. Absorbable cyanoacrylate surgical sealant in kidney transplantation. Transplant Proc. 2011 Sep;43(7):2584-6.

[13] Salehipour M, Salahi H, Fathikalajahi A, Mohammadian R, Emadmarvasti V, Bahador A, Nikeghbalian S, Kazemi K, Dehghani M, Malek-Hosseini SA. Is perioperative intravesically applied antibiotic solution effective in the prophylaxis of urinary tract infections after renal transplantation? Urol Int. 2010;85(1):66-9. Epub 2010 Mar 17

[14] Manassero F, Di Paola G, Mogorovich A, Giannarini G, Boggi U, Selli C. Orthotopic bladder substitute in renal transplant recipients: experience with Studer technique and literature review. Transpl Int. 2011 Sep;24(9):943-8. Epub 2011 Jul 1. Review.

[15] Wagner M, Dieckmann KP, Klän R, Fielder U, Offermann G. Rescue of renal transplants with distal ureteral complications bypyelo-pyelostomy. J Urol. 1994 Mar;151(3):578-81.

[16] Parapiboon W, Ingsathit A, Disthabanchong S, Nongnuch A, Jearanaipreprem A, Charoenthanakit C, Jirasiritham S, Sumethkul V. Impact of early ureteric stent removal and cost-benefit analysis in kidney transplant recipients: results of a randomized controlled study. Transplant Proc. 2012 Apr;44(3):737-9.

[17] Kayler L, Kang D, Molmenti E, Howard R: Kidney transplant ureteroneocystostomy techniques and complications: review of the literature. Transplant Proc. 2010 Jun;42(5): 1413-20.

[18] Schanfield I: New experimental methods for implantation of the ureter in bladder and conduit. Transplant Proc 4:637, 1972

[19] MacKinnon KJ, Oliver JA, Morehouse DD, et al: Cadaver renal transplantation: emphasis on urological aspects. J Urol 99:486, 1968

[20] Barry JM: Unstented extravesical ureteroneocystostomy in kidney transplantation. J Urol 129:918, 1983.

[21] Starzl TE, Shapiro R, Tzakis A, et al: A new technique of extravesical ureteroneocystostomy for renal transplantation. Transplant Proc 21:3856, 1989

[22] Davari HR, Yarmohammadi H, Malek-hosseini SA, Salahi H, Bahador A, Salehipour M. Urological complications in 980 consecutive patients with renal transplantation. Int J Urol. 2006 Oct;13(10):1271-5.

Chapter 2

Renal Aging and Kidney Transplantation

Katrien De Vusser and Maarten Naesens

Additional information is available at the end of the chapter

1. Introduction

Kidney transplantation is the preferred therapy for most patients with end-stage renal disease. The demand for kidney grafts however far exceeds the supply of available organs. As a result, transplant teams increasingly use organs from extended criteria donors, of older age or with significant comorbidity. This use of extended criteria organs is not without consequences.

Older donor age is strongly related to impaired kidney graft function and graft failure because older kidneys are limited in their capacity to tolerate injury [1]. Aging is associated with renal structural changes en functional decline. Older kidneys lose renal parenchyma and trough this have a decreased renal plasma flow and tubular dysfunction. The mechanisms required for tissue repair after damage become less reliable, resulting in a decrease in repair capacity. This functional decline in the potential to repair and regenerate is often considered a hallmark of the aging phenotype [2] [3].

Another major component of the aging phenotype is replicative or cellular senescence, which is defined as permanent, irreversible growth arrest. In this chapter we draw the parallel between the aging kidney in the transplantation setting and cellular senescence.

2. Impact of older donor age on transplantation outcome

The success of organ transplantation in patients with end-stage renal damage gave rise to waiting lists and organ shortage. This in itself led to the increasing use of kidneys from older or expanded criteria donors for transplantation. In 2002 the term Expanded criteria donor (ECD) was codified to be deceased donors aged 60 years of older and those aged 50-59 years with at least 2 of the following characteristics: history of hypertension, serum creatinine level greater than 1.5 mg/dL and cerebrovascular cause of death. The risk of graft failure after an ECD kidney transplant is 70% higher than after a non- ECDtransplant [4].

Also Ojo *et al.* have reported on the survival of recipients of marginal kidneys, defined as kidneys with one or more of the following pretransplant factors: donor age >55 years, non-heartbeating donor, cold ischemia time >36 h, and donor hypertension or diabetes mellitus of >10 years duration. Also in this study, marginal kidney transplants had a lower allograft outcomes compared with organs from ideal donors [5].

In another study, Woo *et al.* compared two groups only divided by age. There was a larger increase in graft failure rates of kidneys from donors >55 years of age. Also the mean estimated glomerular filtration rate 6 months post-transplant and the stability of the glomerular filtration rate in the first transplant year were significantly higher in the recipients of donors <55 years [6].

Recent data on 1063 kidney grafts from living donors confirm the association between older donor age and graft outcome even after living donation, where living donors are screened prior to transplantation and comorbidities are avoided. Increasing living donor age was associated with lower kidney function after transplantation, loss of glomerular filtration rate beyond 1 year and reduced graft survival [7].

With the increasing use of older and extended criteria donor kidneys, the intrinsic quality of the kidneys at transplantation is nowadays much more important for the post-transplant histological evolution and long-term graft survival than acute T-cell mediated rejection [1, 8, 9]. The causes by which older kidneys lose function after transplantation remain however incompletely understood. This may involve both early and late-onset processes and is likely to be found mainly in a significant effect of donor age on the subclinical progression of chronic histological damage [10]. In a large study using protocol biopsies, it was not only demonstrated that higher donor age is the major determinant of this non-specific chronic allograft damage, but also that the association between donor age and post-transplant histological damage is independent of the histological quality of the graft at implantation [11]. This suggests that donor age and the aging process in itself are playing an independent role on renal allograft histological progression and long-term outcome. From these studies, it can even be hypothesized that the aging process in itself is accelerated after transplantation, and contributes to transplant outcome [10].

3. Mechanisms of renal aging

It is essential to distinguish aging from age-related disease. Aging itself is not a disease but seems to be the greatest risk factor for age-related pathology [12]. The altered molecules with aging involve many different pathways, including cell integrity, cellular proliferation, cell transport and energy metabolism. Many of these molecules and processes are not unique to aging and are likely general pathways involved in tissue damage and repair. Aging is a programmed biological process that is associated with small transcriptional differences in many genes, rather than large expression changes in a small number of genes [13-16].

The aging phenotype is the consequence of cellular senescence, of increased susceptibility to apoptosis with older age, of impaired regeneration and repair, of decreased functional capacity of stem cells and progenitor cells, of changes in the expression of growth factors with increasing age, of mitochondrial changes, of dysregulation of autoregulatory pathways and of immune system alterations and different immunogenicity of older tissue.

Of the previously mentioned mechanisms of aging, cellular senescence is classically seen as one of the most important drivers of the aging process. Cellular senescence leads to permanent and irreversible growth arrest and was detected in seminal *in vitro* studies by Hayflick and Moorhead [17, 18]. Senescent cells remain viable but show a changed morphology, greater heterogeneity, expression of SA-β-gal, accumulation of lipofuscin granules and lack of response to mitogenic stimuli.

Cellular senescence is a specific response of mitotically active cells to various stressors. It is determined by multiple factors, including the genetic regulation of metabolism, time, the number cell cycles of replication, and most importantly the answer to injury and stress [11, 19]. Examples of these different factors are telomere shortening and telomere dysfunction, non-telomere DNA damage (e.g. due to X-rays, oxidative stress and UV irradiation), mitogenic signals including those produces by oncogens (wich also cause DNA damage) and non-genotoxic stress like chromatin perturbation (epigenetic changes) and other stress factors [20, 21] (. Cellular senescence thus not only comprises exhaustion of a predetermined proliferative capacity (intrinsic senescence or replicative senescence), but can also be induced by extrinsic factors (stress-induced premature senescence).

In this light, the impact of cellular senescence goes beyond the importance for aging. Cellular senescence pathways play essential roles in tumor suppression, tumor promotion and tissue repair.

There is increasing evidence that cellular senescence is a tumor suppressive system (by inducing growth arrest) and a tumor-promoting phenomenon (by secretion of inflammatory cytokines) [22]. To reconcile the apparently conflicting impact of cellular senescence on cancer, Campisi *et al.* suggest that cellular senescence is a biological process that was selected to promote fitness in young organisms (beneficial: tumor suppression, tissue regeneration), but is deleterious in old organisms (harming: aging, tumor promotion) [23]. In the evolution, senescence pathways evolved in an environment where organism lifespan was short. Therefore tumor-suppressor mechanisms needed to be effective for only a relatively short (reproductive) period [21]. Even if this mechanism was harmful later on, this would not affect selective pressure. This concept is the essence of the "antagonistic pleiotropy hypothesis" and makes us understand the senescence concept much better [23].

4. The replicative senescence pathways in renal disease and transplantation

Replicative senescence depends mainly on two pathways: the ARF-p53-p21 signaling pathway that is partially telomere dependent and the p16-pRb pathway, which is independent of telomere dysfunction. These pathways interact but can act independently [21, 24].

1. Replicative senescence pathways ARF-p53-p21 (associated with telomere shortening).

Telomeres comprise tandem TTAGGG repeats of 5000 to 15000 base pairs that normally reside at the ends of chromosome ends as protection and prevent end-to-end fusion of chromosomes. Telomeric DNA is synthesized and its length is regulated by telomerase. Most somatic cells don't express telomerase and mature telomeres tend to progressively shorten with every cell division. The crucial role of telomerase absence in the telomere shortening is proven *in vitro* as telomere shortening can be bypassed by transfection with telomerase [25].

Telomere length reflects several important factors such as heredity, telomerase activity, the efficiency of telomere-binding proteins, the rate of cellular proliferation and oxidative stress in the milieu. Although telomere length is partly heritable, there are major differences in telomere length even among monozygotic twins, which suggests that environmental factors (e.g. hyperglycemie, oxidative stress [26, 27]) play a major role in telomere attrition and aging.

When the telomeres become critically short (reach the "Hayflick limit") a classical DNA-damage response is triggered with participation of several protein kinases (e.g. ATM and CHK2), adaptor proteins (e.g. 53BP1 and MDC1) and chromatin modifiers (e.g. gammaH2AX). Telomere shortening also leads to activation of the p53 pathway (trough p53 phosphorylation) and herewith associated p21 (also termed CDKN1a, p21Cip1, Waf1 or SD11) expression. Also other DNA damage responses (DDRs) and ARF (alternate reading frame, p14) can lead to activation of the p53 pathway. SIRT1 (sirtuin 1) can negatively regulate p53 localization to the nucleus and its function as a transcription factor.

The clinical importance of telomere shortening has been suggested in a very interesting study, where leukocyte telomere length was used as a biomarker of aging. In this study, the association between telomere length and various disease processes was independent of chronological age, which suggests the value of telomere length measurement as a biomarker of biological or cellular age [28].

In contrast to, e.g. blood cells, the association between age and telomere shortening in renal tissue was only studied scarcely. The supposed association with reduced regenerative capacity during aging and chronic diseases, and after acute injury, seems valid but has never been proven in humans. Only Westhoff's study in telomerase deficient mice suggests that critical telomere shortening in kidneys leads to increased senescence and apoptosis, thereby limiting regenerative capacity [29].

In adult kidneys, telomerase activity is very low, which results in telomere shortening by every cell division, as was demonstrated by Melk *et al* [25]. Also ischemia can induce telomere shortening as has been shown in different animal models [30-32] Finally, glomerular diseases like IgA nephropathy, lupus nephritis and focal glomerulosclerosis are associated with increased p53 expression compared to kidneys without lesions, both in animals [33] and in humans [34, 35] Whether this relates to telomere length has not been studied to date.

After bone marrow transplantation telomere shortening occurs significantly more rapidly than would be expected in graft-derived leukocytes. Probably due to the replicative stress on the blood cell caused the kinetics of haemopoietic engraftment [36]. After solid organ transplantation there are arguments to state that transplantation is associated with accelerated shortening of telomere length in the transplanted cells [12]. In transplanted renal cells, there is evidence for an increased cell turnover at the time of transplantation and a phase of increased cell regeneration directly after transplantation that correlates with cold ischemia time [37, 38]. Also a small study showed that shorter telomere length in biopsies obtained at implantation was associated with lower graft function at 12 months after transplantation, but no correlation with p21 or p53 was found [39]. These studies need further validation to confirm the role of telomere shortening on transplant outcome.

2. p16-pRB pathways (independent of telomere dysfunction).

DNA damage by environmental stress is the main stressor for activation of the p16-pRB pathway although dysfunctional telomeres can also induce p16 [21]. This telomere-independent senescence pathway is currently often referred to as 'STATIS' (Stress and Aberrant Signaling-Induced Senescence. P16 (encoded by *CDKN2A*) is an important tumor suppressor in the p53 pathway. P16 keeps pRB in an active hypophosphorylated form, which inhibits cell proliferation and induces growth arrest [12]. The p53 and p16-pRB pathways interact witch each other and there is a reciprocal regulation.

In native kidneys increased p16 expression is found in human kidneys with glomerular disease [16], interstitial fibrosis, diabetic nephropathy [40] and animal kidneys with hypertension [41]. Furthermore p16 is induced by cyclosporine, catch up growth in low birth weight and is attenuated by calorie restriction [12]. Finally, p16 expression correlates significantly with kidney age [42].

Like the p53 pathway p16 expression relates to ischemia-reperfusion, at least in mice [43]. Furthermore, a rapid increase in p16 expression after transplantation has been described in murine kidney grafts, which was most pronounced in older animals. Whether these findings are also valid in humans, remains unknown.

5. Summary

In summary, there is extensive data that the outcome of kidney transplantation is heavily influenced by the age of the transplanted kidneys. There is some scant evidence that transplantation in itself increases cell turnover and leads to accelerate replicative senescence. Whether the association between older kidneys and impaired graft outcome relates to this accelerate replicative senescence after transplantation is however not clear, and the few suggestions in the literature need to be validated in large-enough patient cohorts.

Author details

Katrien De Vusser and Maarten Naesens

Department of Nephrology and Renal Transplantation, University Hospitals Leuven, Leuven, Belgium

References

[1] Meier-Kriesche, H.U., et al., Lack of Improvement in Renal Allograft Survival Despite a Marked Decrease in Acute Rejection Rates Over the Most Recent Era. Am J Transplant, 2004. 4(3): p. 378-383.

[2] Epstein, M., Aging and the kidney. J.Am.Soc.Nephrol., 1996. 7(8): p. 1106-1122.

[3] Zhou, W., et al., Predominant role for C5b-9 in renal ischemia/reperfusion injury. Journal of Clinical Investigation, 2000. 105(10): p. 1363-1371.

[4] Port, F.K., et al., Donor characteristics associated with reduced graft survival: an approach to expanding the pool of kidney donors. Transplantation, 2002. 74(9): p. 1281-6.

[5] Ojo, A.O., et al., Survival in recipients of marginal cadaveric donor kidneys compared with other recipients and wait-listed transplant candidates. J.Am.Soc.Nephrol., 2001. 12(3): p. 589-597.

[6] Woo, Y.M., et al., The advanced age deceased kidney donor: current outcomes and future opportunities. Kidney Int, 2005. 67(6): p. 2407-2414.

[7] Noppakun, K., et al., Living donor age and kidney transplant outcomes. Am J Transplant, 2011. 11(6): p. 1279-1286.

[8] Summers, D.M., et al., Analysis of factors that affect outcome after transplantation of kidneys donated after cardiac death in the UK: a cohort study. Lancet, 2010. 376(9749): p. 1303-1311.

[9] Opelz, G. and B. Dohler, Influence of immunosuppressive regimens on graft survival and secondary outcomes after kidney transplantation. Transplantation, 2009. 87(6): p. 795-802.

[10] Naesens, M., et al., Donor age and renal P-glycoprotein expression associate with chronic histological damage in renal allografts. J Am Soc Nephrol, 2009. 20(11): p. 2468-80.

[11] Halloran, P.F., A. Melk, and C. Barth, Rethinking chronic allograft nephropathy: the concept of accelerated senescence. J.Am.Soc.Nephrol., 1999. 10(1): p. 167-181.

[12] Naesens, M., Replicative senescence in kidney aging, renal disease, and renal transplantation. Discov Med, 2011. 11(56): p. 65-75.

[13] Weindruch, R., et al., Microarray profiling of gene expression in aging and its alteration by caloric restriction in mice. J Nutr., 2001. 131(3): p. 918S-923S.

[14] Rodwell, G.E., et al., A transcriptional profile of aging in the human kidney. PLoS.Biol., 2004. 2(12): p. e427.

[15] McCarroll, S.A., et al., Comparing genomic expression patterns across species identi-
fies shared transcriptional profile in aging. Nat.Genet., 2004. 36(2): p. 197-204.

[16] Melk, A., et al., Increased expression of senescence-associated cell cycle inhibitor
p16INK4a in deteriorating renal transplants and diseased native kidney. Am J Transplant., 2005. 5(6): p. 1375-1382.

[17] Kawai, T., et al., HLA-mismatched renal transplantation without maintenance immunosuppression. N.Engl.J.Med., 2008. 358(4): p. 353-361.

[18] Hayflick, L. and P.S. Moorhead, The serial cultivation of human diploid cell strains.
Exp.Cell Res., 1961. 25: p. 585-621.

[19] Hayflick, L., Biological aging is no longer an unsolved problem. Ann.N.Y.Acad.Sci.,
2007. 1100: p. 1-13.

[20] Finkel, T., M. Serrano, and M.A. Blasco, The common biology of cancer and ageing.
Nature, 2007. 448(7155): p. 767-774.

[21] Campisi, J. and F.F. dda di, Cellular senescence: when bad things happen to good
cells. Nat.Rev.Mol.Cell Biol., 2007. 8(9): p. 729-740.

[22] Coppe, J.P., et al., Senescence-associated secretory phenotypes reveal cell-nonautono-
mous functions of oncogenic RAS and the p53 tumor suppressor. PLoS.Biol., 2008.
6(12): p. 2853-2868.

[23] Campisi, J., Cellular senescence: putting the paradoxes in perspective.
Curr.Opin.Genet.Dev., 2010.

[24] Collado, M. and M. Serrano, Senescence in tumours: evidence from mice and humans. Nat.Rev.Cancer, 2010. 10(1): p. 51-57.

[25] Melk, A., et al., Telomere shortening in kidneys with age. J Am Soc Nephrol, 2000.
11(3): p. 444-453.

[26] Yoshida, T., et al., ATF3 protects against renal ischemia-reperfusion injury. J Am Soc
Nephrol, 2008. 19(2): p. 217-224.

[27] Avogaro, A., S.V. de Kreutzenberg, and G.P. Fadini, Insulin signaling and life span.
Pflugers Arch., 2010. 459(2): p. 301-314.

[28] Wong, J.M. and K. Collins, Telomere maintenance and disease. Lancet, 2003.
362(9388): p. 983-8.

[29] Westhoff, J.H., et al., Telomere shortening reduces regenerative capacity after acute
kidney injury. J Am Soc Nephrol, 2010. 21(2): p. 327-336.

[30] Joosten, S.A., et al., Telomere shortening and cellular senescence in a model of chronic renal allograft rejection. Am J Pathol., 2003. 162(4): p. 1305-1312.

[31] Kelly, K.J., et al., P53 mediates the apoptotic response to GTP depletion after renal
      ischemia-reperfusion: protective role of a p53 inhibitor. J Am Soc Nephrol, 2003.
      14(1): p. 128-138.

[32] Megyesi, J., et al., The p53-independent activation of transcription of p21 WAF1/
      CIP1/SDI1 after acute renal failure. Am J Physiol, 1996. 271(6 Pt 2): p. F1211-F1216.

[33] Turner, C.M., et al., Increased expression of the pro-apoptotic ATP-sensitive P2X7 re-
      ceptor in experimental and human glomerulonephritis. Nephrol Dial.Transplant,
      2007. 22(2): p. 386-395.

[34] Takemura, T., et al., Proto-oncogene expression in human glomerular diseases. J
      Pathol., 1996. 178(3): p. 343-351.

[35] Qiu, L.Q., R. Sinniah, and S.I. Hsu, Coupled induction of iNOS and p53 upregulation
      in renal resident cells may be linked with apoptotic activity in the pathogenesis of
      progressive IgA nephropathy. J Am Soc Nephrol, 2004. 15(8): p. 2066-2078.

[36] Wynn, R.F., et al., Accelerated telomere shortening in young recipients of allogeneic
      bone-marrow transplants. Lancet, 1998. 351(9097): p. 178-181.

[37] Oberbauer, R., et al., Apoptosis of tubular epithelial cells in donor kidney biopsies
      predicts early renal allograft function. J.Am.Soc.Nephrol., 1999. 10(9): p. 2006-2013.

[38] Vinuesa, E., et al., Macrophage involvement in the kidney repair phase after ischae-
      mia/reperfusion injury. J Pathol., 2008. 214(1): p. 104-113.

[39] Koppelstaetter, C., et al., Markers of cellular senescence in zero hour biopsies predict
      outcome in renal transplantation. Aging Cell, 2008. 7(4): p. 491-497.

[40] Verzola, D., et al., Accelerated senescence in the kidneys of patients with type 2 dia-
      betic nephropathy. AJP - Renal Physiology, 2008. 295(5): p. F1563-F1573.

[41] Westhoff, J.H., et al., Hypertension induces somatic cellular senescence in rats and
      humans by induction of cell cycle inhibitor p16INK4a. Hypertension, 2008. 52(1): p.
      123-129.

[42] Chkhotua, A.B., et al., Increased expression of P21((WAF1/CIP1)) CDKI gene in
      chronic allograft nephropathy correlating with the number of acute rejection epi-
      sodes. Transplant Proc., 2003. 35(2): p. 655-658.

[43] Hochegger, K., et al., p21 and mTERT are novel markers for determining different is-
      chemic time periods in renal ischemia-reperfusion injury. AJP - Renal Physiology,
      2007. 292(2): p. F762-F768.

Chapter 3

Policies and Methods to Enhance the Donation Rates

Lucan Mihai, Lucan Valerian Ciprian and Iacob Gheorghiță

Additional information is available at the end of the chapter

1. Introduction

The therapeutic promise of transplanting organs from cadaveric donors, as envisioned by the pioneers of transplantation, has never been kept because the demand for cadaveric organs has by far exceeded the supply.

Besides the fact that renal transplantation is the optimal treatment for patients with end stage renal disease, it provides benefits to the society as a whole as well as to the recipients. Yet, the donor shortage poses a significant challenge to the transplant community and bare unfavorable consequences: prolonged waiting time and compromise patient survival. Sustained efforts were done during times to increase both the deceased donor and living donor pool.

The expanded criteria donors also known as non-traditional donors has been credited to lessen the current shortage of grafts available for transplantation by providing more grafts. Any such attempt is a two-edged sword since it increases the outcome risk of the suboptimal grafts.

Criteria for living donation were more restrictive compared with cadaver donation but such reluctance to use living donor marginal grafts is declining since transplantation is a better option than dialysis.

Expansion criteria allows transplantation of grafts from deceased donors at the extreme age (above 60 and below 16), with history of hypertension, diabetes or malignancy, hemodynamically unstable, non-heartbeating, seropositive for hepatitis B or C, with systemic infections, at high-risk for HIV infection, reduced renal function, anatomic anomalies, or injuries [1].

The waiting list for transplant organs continues to grow and many patients continues to die while waiting or become unsuitable for organ transplantation. Consequently, many patients with end stage organ failure are no longer relaying on the waiting list for cadaver transplantation. There is a trend not only to reconsider the living donor but also to turn the attention toward spouses, friends or even strangers as possible donors. From medical point of view, all these are acceptable alternatives due to advances in immunosuppression which have eliminated the requirement for a perfect genetic match for a successful organ transplantation. In many US transplant centers, the number of kidneys obtained from living donors has exceeded the number of kidneys obtained from cadaver [2].

Although organs from living donors can be transplanted safely, concerns about the protection of well-being of such donors has prompted the transplantation community to develop a consensus statement, emphasizing that a living donor should be competent, willing to donate an organ, and free of coercion.

Regardless of donor type and graft quality, one should keep in mind that never should be transplanted grafts with a heightened potential for the development of a progressive disease.

Since the rules are continuously evolving, the approach to use of each graft and recipient selection should be done with caution in order to obtain acceptable results.

2. The living donor

The use of living donors for renal transplantation was critical for the early development of the field, and in fact, preceded the use of cadaveric donors. At the moment, 20-22% of all kidney transplants performed in the world were done with grafts from living donors. Most donors are related genetically to the recipient, but there is an increasing percentage of cases, where donors are genetically unrelated and includes spouses, friends, or other emotionally related individuals. As it is known, ethical guidelines mandate that the living donors should not be coerced and there will be no evidence of financial profit for the donor. As a consequence, the donation should be considered "a gift of extraordinary value". It is known that the use of living donors has been associated with a higher success rate than that seen with cadaveric donation. Due to a higher demand for transplantation and the lack of a parallel increase in the number of available cadaveric organs, living donation is the only solution for some patients to avoid long times on waiting list, and occasionally, even the need of dialysis (1).

Better results (both long and short-term)
Consistent early function and easier management
Avoidance of long waiting time for transplantation
Less aggressive immunosuppressive regimens
Emotional gain to donor

Table 1. Advantages of living donation

There is a remote risk of catastrophic outcome of the living donor (1 in 3200 patients), but most transplant centers and surgeons accept this. Some centers accept only living related donors; others accept related as well as unrelated donors. These centers come to turns with the possibility of harming living donors by being highly selective in their acceptance of donors. While surgically pragmatic, there is a philosophic fallacy in this approach. The important issues regarding the donor, in addition to medical suitability, are whether the donor understands the risk of nephrectomy and whether the donor freely consents. The risk for the donor is the same regardless of the donor's relationship to the recipient and regardless of the recipient's outcome. The risk for the surgeon, that is the death of the donor, is no less devastating for the surgeon if the patient is a close relative to the recipient than if the donor is a stranger.

2.1. Evaluation of the living donor

Usually, the potential living donor is the one who initiates the discussion about donation, although the recipient or the physician can also rise the issue. The donor than meets with the nephrologist, transplant surgeon, social worker, and transplant coordinator. All donors are informed of the risks and benefits of the transplantation compared with the dialysis and the risks to themselves by donating a kidney, on both short and long term [3, 4]. 1995 data of US practices founded that reported mortality rate for living donors to be 0.03% and the morbidity rate to be 0.23%. It is important to screen any relative of a patient with familial renal disease (polycystic kidney disease, hereditary nephritis) for evidence of occult signs and symptoms, in order to exclude such donors [5]. On the other hand, kidneys with minor renal abnormalities can be used safely, once it is determined that function of the such kidneys could not be impaired after transplantation [6].

Initial evaluation of all potential donors consists of blood and tissue typing. Usually, those with ABO incompatibility are excluded; compatibility with the Rh factor is unnecessary. All blood group compatible donors are then tested with the T lymphocyte cross-match. A negative cross-match will allow further consideration for donation. In the case of multiple potential donors, the better the antigen match, the grater is the likelihood of being selected for donation, if all other testing are within normal limits. In general, as long as the donor and the recipient have a negative T cell cross-match, the operation can be cared out. This is true for both related and non-related donors who are ABO compatible. Many centers perform a mixed lymphocyte reaction (MLR) as part of the routine evaluation, but the importance of this test has decreased with the introduction of better immunosuppression.

Further evaluation for a potential donor consist of a complete medical history and a complete physical examination, routine laboratory, testing, and serologic evaluation for EBV, herpes virus, CMV, HIV, and hepatitis B and C viruses. Urinalysis and culture along with 24 hour urine collection for creatinine clearance and protein excretion, are included as part of the routine evaluation. If there is any concern regarding a borderline hypertensive pressure reading, the blood pressure should be measured on the least three and as many as ten separate occasions. Once all laboratory testing has been performed, the next step is renal arteriography with an excretion faze to visualize the collecting system. This eliminate the need for intravenous pyelography. Such testing can be performed on an outpatient basis. Nowadays spiral CT scan has been used routinely instead of conventional angiography in all centers. The use of magnetic resonance (MR) angiography is also growing in importance. Donors are judged unsuitably for a variety of reasons (2).

Absolute
Lack of discernment
Alcohol or drug addiction
Age less than 18 years
Hypertension: blood pressure over 140/90 mm Hg requiring medication
Diabetes: abnormal glucose tolerance test or HbA1c
Proteinuria: over 300 mg/24 hours
Abnormal glomerular filtration rate: creatinine clearance less than 75 mL/min.
Microscopic hematuria of unexplained cause
History of thrombosis or thrombembolism
Medical significant illness: chronic lung disease, recent malignant tumor, heart disease, vascular collagen disease,
History of bilateral kidney stones
Family history of autosomal dominant polycystic kidney disease (ADPKD), unless ultrasound or CT scan is normal and age is over 30 years
Familial history of renal cancer
Bilateral fibromuscular arterial dysplasia
Long-term use of nephrotoxic drugs
HIV positive
Hepatitis B antigen-positive to a negative recipient or unprotected
Other severe infections

Relative
Anatomic abnormalities of the donor's kidney: vascular or urological
Obesity: 30% or more above ideal weight
Young donor with a first degree relative with type I diabetes or renal disease
Significant previous abdominal surgery
Single history of unilateral renal stone disease
ABO incompatible
Positive cross-match
Smoking
Psychiatric disorders

Table 2. Exclusion criteria for living donors

Anyone at risk for the development of acquired renal disease should be excluded. This includes individuals with diastolic blood pressure constantly above 90 mm Hg, or who required hypertensive medication to control their blood pressure.

History of hypertension is not by itself a reason for exclusion if the donor is normotensive and off medication, but the donor should be carefully examined for preexisting renal disease or for the risk of development of renal disease later in life.

Potential donors for siblings with diabetes routinely undergo a five hours glucose tolerance test, and 24 hour urine specimen must be free of proteinuria. Some centers require that the donor be at least 10 years older than the age of the recipient at the time of diagnosis of the diabetes. The measurement of the haemoglobin A1c and anti-islet antibodies also can be included in the evaluation of any potential related living donor for a recipient with diabetes. Unexplained microscopic hematuria may be an indication of an underlying renal disease such as glomerulonephritis, but it may not be detected before donation. Finding as few as three red cells per high power field may appear unimportant at first but may be an indicator of potential future problems.

History of thrombembolism or thromboflebitis places the potential donor at increased risk of pulmonary embolism and therefore it precludes donation. This is also true for patients with heart disease, or history of malignant neoplasia. Obesity may be a relative contraindication for any potential donor, if it is more than 30% above ideal body weight. These individuals should be advised to loose the excess body weight before the transplant is scheduled, to decrease the risk of pulmonary embolism or cardiac complications.

Patients with clinically significant psychiatric disorders should be fully evaluated by a psychiatrist to established that the donor understands and agrees to the proposed procedure.

Once a full evaluation has been performed, if examination of the donor's kidney vascular supply and drainage system reveals an abnormality, it must be decided whether the risk imposed on the donor or the recipient are too great. With regard to vascular abnormalities we tend to use donor kidneys with three or more arteries if there is a good immunological correspondence and a strong determination for donation and if dialysis tolerance of the recipient is bad [7,8]. Abnormalities such as aneurisms, renal artery stenosis, fibro-muscular dysplasia, if limited in sized and area, can often be resected, repaired, or excised on the back table. Such pathological addition should bee limited to one kidney, living as a rule, the normal kidney in place. Given this caveats, it may be possible to use such donors [9].

Excision and reconstruction of such abnormalities is, in a sense, a of form of treatment of this donors, although care must be taken to avoid living either the donor or the recipient with less than a perfect outcome.

2.2. Preoperative management

Once the evaluation has demonstrated that there are no abnormalities serious enough to exclude donation, the donor can be admitted to the hospital after a spiral CT scan was performed. Many insurance companies are now restricting admissions to the day of the operation. In such cases intravenous hydration can be given overnight on an outpatient basis, or started on arrival at the hospital. Such hydration is important to help ensure adequate diuresis during the donor operation. Preoperative assessment by the anesthesiologist and the pain management team can make for a more comfortable postoperative recovery.

The donor is instructed preoperatively on the use of spirometer, and on the use of leg support stockings and the sequential compression device system to prevent venous stasis. After entering the operating room and before the incision, the patient should receive a dose of intravenous antibiotic. Although preoperative skin cleaning is recommended; hair clipping is avoid until just before incision.

2.3. Surgical alternatives in life donor nephrectomy

Regarding the surgical habits and the existing experience, there are several ways of harvesting kidneys from living donors [10-12].

- Classic transperitoneal approach, either throw midline, or throw a left or right subcostal incision.

- Subcostal extraperitoneal approach (left or wright).

- Dorsal lumbotomy approach. The incision can be performed either underneath the XIIth rib, resecting the XIIth rib, or above the XIIth rib (extraperitoneal, extrapleural).

- Laparoscopic approach either transperitoneal or retroperitoneoscopic.

2.4. Laparoscopic approach for living donor nephrectomy

The introduction of laparoscopic living kidney donation has been a major advance in organ donation. First introduced with some reticence only in selected centers, this procedures are now the preferred surgical approach in almost all transplant programs in United States and Europe. Usually, the program that offers this kind of procedure have a high rates of living kidney donation. The major benefit of laparoscopic technique includes significant reduction of surgical pain, postoperative convalescence, and recovery time. As a result, the laparoscopic donor nephrectomy has been responsible for expanding the pool of living donors and may account for the increased popularity and frequency of living donation. Long term renal function is not different between open nephrectomy and laparoscopic nephrectomy. About 75% of living donor transplant nephrectomies world wide employ laparoscopic technique, either transperitoneal or retroperitoneal.

2.5. Open living donor nephrectomy

The traditional method for removing kidney from a living donor has been open surgical technique, in majority of cases using a flank incision. In selected cases in which the donor has motivation which precluded laparoscopic access (e.g. significant prior abdominal surgery), or in some cases of complex vascular anatomy, an open surgical approach is preferred. Some centers advocate the use of open surgery for pediatric patients, although the age of recipient is not universally considered an indication for open renal procurement. Most donor surgeon use a donor flank incision, extra pleural and extra peritoneal above or below the XIIth rib.

As it is in any surgical approach, the kidney must be very carefully dissected to preserve renal veins and periureteral blood supply. Excessive pressure on the renal artery is avoided to prevent a vasospasm. After the renal vessels are securely ligated and divided the kidney is removed and placed in a basin of frozen saline slush to decrease the renal metabolism and after that the vessels are un-ligated and flushed with heparinized solution for both procedures, either laparoscopic harvesting or classic surgery.

2.6. Postoperative care

Postoperative care of a living donor is fairly standard. Adequate postoperative analgesia is a key factor including postoperative complications such atelectasia and pneumonia [15]. Infections should not occur with appropriate antibiotic prophylaxis. The continuous use of leg stoching and sequential compression devices are essential to prevent deep venous thrombosis of the lower limb. Most patients are often ambulatory by postoperative day 1 or 2 and tolerating oral feedings by postoperative day 2 or 3. The donor can be discharged by postoperative day 2 to 6. The renal function of the donor should be assessed periodically after the operation, as some patients experience a 25% increase in serum creatinine level; this should return near baseline by 3 months after the operation. In fact there are no convincing data to suggest that living donors are at any increased long term risk as a result as having donating the kidney.

2.7. Long term complications

The immediate operative risk to the donor can be stated with some certainty but the long terms effects are not completely understood. Follow-up, in general, is reassuringly but incomplete. Most folow-up studies of living kidney donors find no decrease in long term survival. All existing follow-up found an at least 85% survival up to 31 year after donation, compared to a predicted 66% in general population of similar age. The survival advantage at the living donors was attributed to the selection bias of only healthy individual as renal donors and at better follow up for them. Concerns regarding the possibility that donors will develop end stage renal disease (ESRD) is:

• hyper filtration in the remaining kidney will lead to focal segmental glomerulosclerosis and renal failure, that is donation per se will cause renal failure,

• the second concern is that donor will develop primary renal disease. The donors who develop primary renal disease will progress to renal failure more quickly because they have a lower than normal renal mass at onset of a primary renal disease. The later concern applies to a family with a history that put them for a risk of renal disease, for example: patient with type II diabetes.

Many follow-up studies have noted an increase in hypertension and proteinuria as well as a statistically but not clinically significant increase in serum creatinine. There are studies which found an increase in 20% of patients with blood pressure (15%-48%) [16] but it is not clear if hypertension is more common to this group than in general population.

Another study is finding that 35% of patients are taking anti-hypertensive medications and 23% are having proteinuria compared with 44% and 22% respectively for controls [17]. On the other side, even if the donor has a normal renal function, the glomerular filtration rate is in fact maintained by hyper filtration.

One thing is for sure, that in all follow-up studies, majority of the donors which are altruistic donors, drive a tremendous degree of satisfaction and an increased of self esteem for their donation. As a consequence, donors interviewed considered their donation as an act of heroism and generosity with which nothing else in their life can be compared [18]. More than 90% said that they would donate if they have it to do over again, and fewer than 10% expressed any regret about donating [19].

2.8. Policies to enhance living donation

The therapeutic promise of transplanting organs from cadaveric donors has never been kept because the demand for transplantation has by far exceeded the possibilities. The waiting list for transplants continues to grow and in 2005 nearly 5000 patients were removed from the waiting list because of the death. Consequently many patients with end stage organ failure are no longer relaying on waiting list. Than the attention was turning toward living donors others than they have been classically admitted i.e. toward spouses, friends, or even strangers, as possible donors. From medical point of view, these are acceptable alternatives, due to the fact that immunosuppression has eliminated the requirement for a perfect genetic match in order to have a successful transplantation [20]. In many centers world wide, specially US transplantation centers and scandinavian transplant centers, the number of kidneys transplanted from living donors has exceeded the number of kidneys obtained from cadaver donors (over 35%) [21].

Although donors from living donors can be transplanted safely, concerns about the protection of well being of donors has prompted the transplantation community to develop a consensus statement emphasizing that a living donor should be competent, willing to donate an organ, and free of any kind of coercion [22]. More than that, the new reliance on organs from living donor has increased the risk of donation for financial reasons, especially in the case of unrelated donor. It is world-wide admitted that organ donation has to rely on the voluntarism and altruism, and uncompensated family members of the donor.

Donor type	1990	2000	2010	relative ratio
Cadaveric	4306	5489	7241	+ 1,68
Biologically related living donors	1831	4030	3046	+ 1,66
Emotionally related living donors	59	667	715	+ 12,11
Unrelated living donors	204	804	2516	+ 12,33
Total transplants	6400	10990	13518	+ 2,11

Table 3. Reported kidney transplants performed in USA [OPTN data]

The purchase of organs is explicitly unlawful in Europe, US, as virtually all other countries but the shortage of cadaveric organs has led to a world-wide black market for organs from living donors. That's why patients with sufficient means can travel to distant locations in order to purchase kidneys for transplantation [23, 24].

This is a dramatic situation which is generated by continuous shortage of organs for transplantation and by the increasingly donation rate from unrelated living donors. Such a situation require significant changes in the transplantation laws which should permit the increase of living donors and in the same time to stop the organ trade. Very difficult task.

The rate of living donation can be increased by two methods:

• organizing and ethic alternatives,

• medical methods are represented by: laparoscopic harvesting, paired kidney exchange, transplantation of grafts with anatomic abnormalities (vascular, urinary tract or fusion), acceptance of patients with low compatibility after a treatment with plasmapheresis and iv Ig.

2.8.1. Organizing and ethic alternatives to increase the rate of living donation

The motives of living donors and the motives of families of deceased donors, are complex and not necessarily always pure altruistic [25]. Spouses and siblings, who act as a living donor, experience a personal reward seeing that the recipient well being is restored. Because the organ donation is a voluntary and valuable act it should be considered as a charitable gift. Society could explicitly thank the organ donors for their gift, as it is done with other charitable contributions, without jeopardizing its altruistic basis. New legislations should embrace ethically acceptable ways to encourage such charitable donation of organs.

2.8.1.1. Incentives for organ donation

The issue of public incentives to enhance donation is more than just complex but mainly sensitive. From a philosophical point of view, the body is a part of our personality, thus in respect with human dignity it would be wrong to use parts of our body as means only [26]. On the other hand, one may assert that everyone is the rightful owner of his person supporting the idea that the self can decide over its body like any kind of property [27].

Most frequently, the background attitude of general population is to reject incentives for donation but there might be circumstances under which attitudes may change [28]. For instance, when the process became transparent: the amount of compensations are specified or there might be some ethical reasons to do so. The main risk is exploitation of those severe impoverished on a black market [29].

The valuable exchange of organs is prohibited worldwide, yet there exists national law or regulations which allows incentives for deceased or living donation [30]. Such incentives including financial reimbursement, health care-related reimbursement or other recognition for living donors or deceased donors' families have been widely debated [31].

Donor medal of honor. Organ procurement organizations must have ceremonies which recognize and appreciate organ donation. A donor medal of honor enacted by a top official of the country expresses the appreciation and gratitude on behalf of the whole community to the living donors and even to the families of the deceased donor [32, 33].

Medical leave for organ donation. Currently organ donors risk loss of wages or even loss of employment because the time away from the work that is required for donation [34,35]. In many countries there are legislations that provide a 30 day medical leave for all employees who donate an organ for transplantation [36]. However, no one should have to incur a personal expense for donating an organ. Many national organizations are doing an effort to encourage hospitals with transplantation services to provide paid medical leave for employees who become organ donors. Even if legislation emphasizing that enrichment should not be the reason for the donation, paid medical leave has to be available to a larger number of would-be donors [37].

Ensuring access to organs for previous donors. As you have seen up to now, the majority of living donors are doing well after donation. However, it has been established that at 10 years after donation, under 5% of those who donated the kidney developed ESRD; this donors are being placed on waiting list for cadaver organs [38]. Despite the additional allocation priority points, these donors have to wait for a cadaveric kidney, some of them for a long period of time. The health and well being of living donor should be monitored in a follow-up register in order to document medical problems associated with donation that occur over ensuing years [22]. The need for a transplant in a previous kidney donor should be considered a high priority in the allocation of the organs.

Donor insurance. The fact that there are being cases in which a kidney donor died immediately after donation or needed a kidney transplant at a later date, serves as a reminder that a nephrectomy (any kind of nephrectomy) is not a risk free procedure. A survey at some centers of transplantation show that at least two kidney donors had died from perioperative complications after a kidney donation and some of them had a persistent complication [39].

As a consequence, it should be enacted national plans to provide life and disability ensures for all living donors including a mechanism to ensure that they do not incur catastrophic medical expenses as a result of a donation.

2.8.1.2. Organ exchanges

Since the report of Rapaport which introduced the concept of paired kidney exchange as a method to enhance the number of living donors, these techniques have been applied in several countries with lower cadaver donation rates like Mexico, South Korea, Japan, and Europe (Holland and Romania).

Many persons who wished to donate an organ to a spouse or another family member where unable to help them due to incompatible blood type or other immunological barriers (positive cross-match). A program of paired kidney exchange addresses this problem by permitting an exchange of organs from two living donors [34] or from one living donor to one deceased donor. In the later approach, recently introduced in New England and Holland, a living donor incompatible with his intending recipient, donates an organ to a compatible patient on the waiting list for cadaveric organs in exchange for a priority allocation of a cadaveric organ to the donor's intended recipient. Thus, two transplantations are performed in circumstances that otherwise had permitted neither. Because such exchange could open the door to a paid donorship, the same prohibition against the payment donor should be applied to organ exchanges.

Legal issues. Initially, most countries limited traditional transplantation to genetically of strong emotionally related pairs. With extend of paired kidney donation, such limitations were removed to allow both altruistic non-directed donation and paired donation. Although, any exchange in paired donation represent in fact a transaction between parts, it do not involve financial values. It is advisable that such a issue should be explicitly addressed by the legal framework of every country.

Allocation algorithm. Grafts allocation in paired kidney donation is one of the domain who largely benefits from theories derived from economics regarding stable allocation and the practice of market design [40]. The main goal is to maximize the number of matched pairs. Any such program should overcome the disadvantage of O recipients by increasing the likelihood to receive a compatible graft. The risk of a positive cross-match with a from the donor pool might be assessed by considering the HLA antibody profile of the recipients and the HLA profile of the donors [41, 42]. When done on a national scale, such a matching should include distance between transplant centers, matching the virusologic profile of the recipient and donor, donor's age and size. Recipients from such pairs will be suspended from the waiting list until either they will be transplanted or a incompatibility test will reveal that the exchange is not possible. List paired donation may increase the rate of transplants by expanding the donor pool. In such an exchange, an incompatible donor who will donate to a recipient from the waiting list while his recipient will receive a high priority for the allocation for a deceased donor kidney [43, 44]. There are several concerns regarding ethical and legal issues. Such a transplant is designed to give an alternative to O blood type recipients with a non-O incompatible donor. The immediate consequence is the transplantation of a non-O blood group recipient from the waiting list and the addition of a O blood group recipient. This way, there will be an increased pressure over the O blood group recipients [43, 44].

Matching algorithms. Different matching algorithms were designed to maximize the number of recipients with an incompatible living donor will undergo renal transplantation. After an initial experience with two pairs, the number of pairs involved in a paired kidney transplantation increases to three, four and even more and the procedure gain worldwide acceptance. Involving of more than two pairs increases the chances to get a renal transplant but in order to avoid the withdrawal risk requires six or more operations to be done at the same time. Designed for O blood group recipients, exchanging of an incompatible kidney for a preferential position on the waiting list increases the recipient's chances for a renal transplantation but decreases the chances of other O blood group recipients from the waiting list [45-48]. This situation creates ethic dilemmas. Generalizing such list exchanges to any blood group recipient with a living donor available but incompatible, may overcome this issue.

Altruistic donation or non-directed donation is more ethical and legal challenging. It is difficult to believe and understand that a good Samaritan really exists and even when exists, national law framework should allow transplantation from unrelated living donor. Altruistic donors may be allocated to a waiting list or to initiate an open chain of paired transplantations [46,49].

Utilizing living donors may decrease the pressure for renal transplantation. Moreover, implementing of different types of kidney exchange could give further solutions to increase the transplantation rates. Combining different approaches to kidney exchange may create complex and versatile solutions to the incompatibility issue, even finding a better match for compatible pairs.

2.8.2. Medical methods to increase the number of living donation

2.8.2.1. Acceptance of grafts with anatomic anomalies

The number of donations can be increased by accepting donors with anatomic anomalies (multiples arteries, multiple veins, moderate dysfunction of the UPJ, renal cyst, complete duplicate ureteral system, solitary stone) which can be corrected in bench surgery.

Anatomical anomalies of the kidney have been considered for a long time as an absolute contraindication for living donation. Even now, many nephrological centers are including in their exclusion criteria for live related or unrelated donation items like urological abnormalities in donors or history or presence of any kidney stones.

But in our days, the majority of transplant centers with experience in the field, due to the shortage of the living donors pool, are considering the contraindication for using grafts with anatomical anomalies just a relative contraindication. Occasionally, the donor has minor unilateral abnormalities such as a renal cyst, ureteropelvic junction obstruction, solitary stones, duplex ureteral system, etc. If the related donor with a good immunological correspondence with the recipient has an abnormal kidney and is the only one available and the evolution of the recipient on hemodialysis is unacceptable, it is advisable to transplant the abnormal kidney, living the donor with the best one.

2.8.2.2. Acceptance of donors with multiple arteries and veins

The management of multiple renal arteries (MRA) are considered technically demanding in renal transplantation programs with kidneys from related or unrelated living donors. Some programs consider the use of multiple arteries and veins as a relative contraindication, because of increased risk of vascular and urological complications.

In addition, the rapidly increasing laparoscopic kidney donation has been accompanied by a significant shift in surgical practice [50,51]. Many centers which are performing laparoscopic harvesting restrict it to the left kidney [52-54]. The limitation to the left kidney leads to a higher utilization rate of kidneys with multiple arteries; in the literature, incidence of unilateral multiple renal arteries is between 18% and 30%, unless one limits laparoscopic nephrectomy only to the kidney with normal anatomy which is precluding 30% of all donors.

By accepting grafts with multiple renal arteries, one may theoretically accept an adverse effect on the outcome of those grafts. Previous authors [55,56], stated that MRA in their reconstruction were associated with several post-transplant complications. This is the motivation why such anatomy was considered to be a transplant contraindication. The most frequent vascular complications which were encountered in reconstruction of multiple arteries were graft thrombosis, stenosis of the renal artery, and an increased risk of reno-vascular hypertension [55-57]. The most frequently ureteral complication encountered [58] were ureteral necrosis and pelvi-caliceal fistulas.

Smaller arteries are more prone to develop premature atherosclerotic occlusion. If that happens with a small accessory lower pole artery it would lead to ischemic distal ureteral stricture.

Any way, recent data collected from the centers and program of renal transplantation with experience in the field, display above any doubt that procurement of kidneys with multiple renal arteries can be accomplished safely and not impose additional medical, social, economical or postoperative clinical evolution burden, on the donor and the recipient.

Overall intraoperative and early postoperative complications of the recipients are not significantly different from the evolution of the recipients who received grafts with single arteries. A low rate of vascular complications is achieved using standard microvascular reconstruction technique with or without autologous vein patches [59-61] or extension graft. More than that, early graft function assessed by urine output and serum creatinine measurements were not significantly different among grafts with single arteries or grafts with multiple reconstructed arteries. In addition, long term quality of function, rejection, graft loss rates and graft survival were also similar. More than that, overall graft survival rates of this patients is exceeding 90% at 3 years.

In summary, the introduction of laparoscopic donor nephrectomy has significantly increased the number of grafts with multiple renal artery. Utilization of this donors, increase the rate of donation with 30% in specific centers. Modern techniques based on microsurgery have reduced dramatically incidence of above mentioned complications. From a patient outcome based perspective, this change in practice showed to be safe for both donors and recipients.

2.8.2.3. Laparoscopic donor nephrectomy - alternative to increase the rate of living donation

One great potential means for obtaining more kidneys is throw live donation. When compared with cadaveric renal transplantation, living donor transplantation has several advantages, in fact well known, which includes better graft survival, more rapid renal function after transplantation, shorter hospitalization and finally lower cost. However, several barriers exists for potential living donors. Significant time is involved when one donates a kidney. Many individuals do not have adequate financial and social support available that would allow them to make a personal sacrifice and a time commitment necessary for kidney donation. Moreover, the relatively prolonged convalescence can have significant financial impact on donor. Finally, fear of pain as well cosmetic concerns, associated with flank incision, can militate against kidney donation.

Laparoscopic living donor nephrectomy (LLDN) with all its alternatives (transperitoneal approach, retroperitoneal approach, hand assisted laparoscopic nephrectomy) was introduced in 1995 by Ratner and Kavoussi [62].

Laparoscopic nephrectomy is more technically demanding than other standard abdominal laparoscopic procedures. The surgeon experience is crucial for minimizing potential morbidity. Significant operative differences are between open and laparoscopic donor nephrectomy. The later approach requires a different set of technical skills than that associated with traditional open surgery. The endoscopic video image is only two dimensional and much narrower when compared with direct vision afforded by open surgery. The types of instrumentation available for working throw the small incision afford only restricted degrees of freedom when compared to the human hand. Moreover, the tactile sensation, currently can not be transmitted through the instrument. The differences are giving a longer operative time with one or even two hours when compared with open donation. All these drawbacks are only partially eliminated by robotic surgery, even if now there is a three dimensional vision of operative field and the mobility of the working instruments is better than that of human hand.

Even so, laparosccopic renal donation and robotic laparoscopic harvesting offers both introperatively and postoperatively great benefits to the donor.

Due to magnification provided by the optical system and the video camera, in experienced hands, the dissection of the renal pedicle is more accurate and if it is realized through retroperitoneal approach it is much more direct and quicker than classical approach.

The decreased size of the incision for extracting kidney and placement of that incision in the lower abdomen, significantly reduce postoperative pain when compared with traditional opened surgery; it also reduce traumatism of the abdominal wall, which is followed by a quicker and better healing and mobilization postoperatively and quicker reintegration of the patient in society.

Usually, these patients resume their oral intake in the first postoperative day and normal alimentation in maximum two days after surgery.

All retrospective comparisons between open and laparoscopic kidney donation show that analgesic requirements for LLDN and robotic LDN, were 30% lower than those for open procedures. Need for oral pain medication is also reduced.

Return to physical demanding work also occurs, on average, 17th days sooner for the laparoscopic group compared with classic operation.

Recipient and graft survival. All retrospective review of the recipient who received a kidney through laparoscopic or robotic laparoscopic donation compared with those who received kidney via standard open nephrectomy shows no statistical differences if the groups are matched in regard with the number of HLA mismatches, donor relationship, diabetes, previous transplant, gender, or race.

Allograft function. The majority experience in the field attest that all grafts functioned intraoperatively and no clinical significant injury occurred to the graft.

	Laparoscopic	Open	P value
Estimated blood loss (mL)	266+/-174	393+/-335	0.027
Operative time (min.)	232+/-33	183+/-27	<0.001
Hospital stay (days)	3.0+/-0.9	5.7+/-1.7	<0.001
Analgesia (days of use)			
Oral narcotics	4	12	<0.001
Acetaminophen	3	17	<0.001
Resumed oral intake (days)	0.8+/-0.5	2.6+/-1.0	<0.001
Returned to work (weeks)	4.0+/-2.3	6.4+/-3.1	0.003

Table 4. Open versus laparoscopic donor nephrectomy

Allograft rejection. The pneumoperitoneum and retropneumoperitoneum reduces renal blood flow and urine output. The potential for ischemia can make the donor kidney more allogenic by inducing MHC class II expression. This problem could be avoided giving donors intraoperatively a 6-8 liters of crystalloid to promote brisk diuresis, and having an accurate dissection of the renal pedicle and harvesting the kidney only in full diuresis. Biopsy proved rejection in laparoscopically obtained kidney occurred in 30% of cases compared with 35.4% of cases of kidneys harvested by open procedure. At 12 months, creatinine clearance in recipient of kidney from laparoscopic and open procedure were both 66 mL/min. (p = not significant).

Laparoscopic nephrectomy gives less postoperative pain, quicker convalescence, better cosmetic results when compared with traditional open operation. In experienced hands, this procedure is accomplished without increasing the risks to donor safety and allograft function. Complications are comparable to those reported in historic series using open surgery. Longer operative time and the need of disposable equipment result in greater hospital costs. However, quicker convalescence permit patients to resume activities sooner and produce market cost savings both for patients and employer.

2.8.2.4. HLA sensitized and ABO incompatible donor and recipient

During the past decade, several innovative protocols have been adopted to overcome transplantation across a positive cross-match or an ABO blood group barrier. Protein A immunoadsorbtion, high dose intravenous immunoglobuline (IVIG), low dose iv Ig in combination with plasmapheresis, rituximab, splenectomy, all of them alone or in combination, can abrogate a positive cross-match and enhance the chance of a highly sensitized patients to receive a cross-match negative organ. Similar strategies can be used for ABO incompatible donors and are particularly effective when the titter of blood group antigen is low.

Plasmapheresis and intravenous immunoglobuline as a rescue therapy for a positive cross-match live donor kidney transplants. The positive cross-match can present a virtually an insurmountable barrier to kidney transplantation. Anti HLA antibodies have been identified as the predominant cause of early graft failure from hyperacute rejection and acute humoral rejection.

Once the consequence of performing a transplant, in the face of a circulating donor specific alloantibody were fully appreciated and routine pre-transplant cross-matching emerged as a standard, hyperacute rejection became rare, but a large population of a highly sensitized patients who have a little hope of receiving transplant has been subsequently identified.

Some of the longest waiting times for a kidney transplant are observed in patients who are allo-sensitized because of a prior transplant, blood transfusions or pregnancy. Some of these recipients have live donor, meet standards criteria for living donor transplantation, but have a positive cross-match with their donor. A combination of plasmapheresis and IVIG under the cover of standard doses of calcineurin inhibitors or rituximab, together with mycophenolate mofetil and steroids, can effectively and durably remove donor specific anti-HLA antibody, preemptively desensitize the recipient who had positive cross-matches with a potential live donor, allowing the transplantation of this patients using a live donor without cases of hyperacute rejection [63].

This preemptive therapy is initiated several weeks before a planned live donor transplant. Our standard protocol was designed to include oral immunosuppressants before first plasmapheresis treatment followed by a maximum six plasmapheresis on alternate days. The recipients, also received seven days of IVIG (100 mg/kg/day).

Cross-over transplantation and paired kidney exchange as a method to fill the gap of positive cross-match and ABO incompatibility. The gap between the number of donors and number of patients waiting for a kidney transplant continues to widen. Fewer patients get transplants every year because of the organ shortage. This patients can receive a donor from a living donor such a family member, a friend, or even a foreign individual.

The pool of such kidneys has not been fully utilized because not all living donors are compatible with their recipient. Patients with available living donor continue dialysis and many of them die because of ABO incompatibility, cross-match positive, low HLA-matching. Since the report made by Rapaport, when was set the bases of kidney exchange between two donor-recipient pairs in order to obtain a better compatibility, things have changed [64-66]. A spouse donor would give her kidney to an unrelated recipient who matched her blood type. That recipient's mate would provide a kidney for the donor's ill spouse. This swap would imply more than two pairs in order to obtain best compatibility. A cross-over renal transplantation or a paired kidney exchange transplantation is defined by a living kidney donation or a living kidney cadaver pool donation and exchange between two or more such couples who are hindered by ABO incompatibility or positive cross-match to give the kidneys not to the own recipients but solve the problem by cross-exchange the kidney between the pairs to make more matches.

The most frequent reason for ABO incompatibility, preventing living donors from donating is a blood group A or B donor and a blood group O recipient. There are many vice-versa pairs but the problem is that the blood group O donors are universal donors for all blood groups. They can give the kidney directly to their recipients than rather to a stranger. When the cross-match is positive with own one's recipient, but this recipient has a negative cross-match with blood group A or B donor from another couple, the problem is solved by exchanging the kidneys between these pairs. Another reason for kidney exchange is when the O to A or B pair get a better HLA matching from 6 miss-matches to 0-3 miss-matches by swapping the kidney with a A or B to O pair.

The pairs involved in a paired exchange program are interviewed to exclude any coercion of the donor, they are informed about the advantage and the risk of the living donation and the informed consent is obtained. Beside that, all donors undergo psychological evaluation.

The inclusion criteria pursued the goal of exchanging equivalent kidneys with equivalent size, anatomy, similar renal function and similar age. The donor are assessed preoperatively by high resolution iv pyelograms, quantitative renal scan and spiral CT scan or MRI. As a general rule, the donors accept to join this program as this is the only way to help their relatives or friends. The transplants involving two or three pairs can be performed simultaneously excepting the session with more than three pairs when the transplants are performed succes-sively. All the transplants are performed by the same surgical team in respect to the principle to equivalent quality of the surgical act.

The basic principle of kidney exchange is the equivalent exchange. To accomplished this, high resolution preoperative work-ups required and unpredicted situation which can hinder harvesting are avoided. This way, simultaneously harvesting is not mandatory.

By using kidney exchange, the recipient benefit from the better matching as well as the known advantages of living donation. Paired kidney exchange reduce the duration of dialysis before transplantation and expand the pool of living donors.

In the countries where the living donation is the main source of organs, cross-over transplan-tation may become more popular as it increase the number of transplants. The kidney exchange program has to be promoted as it offers solutions where apparently there is none.

Transplantation of ABO incompatible pairs. Developed initially in countries with predominant living donation, transplantation of a ABO incompatible kidney is a demanding task but it was possible mainly due to development of more potent immunosuppressive drugs which reduces the risk of hyperacute rejection [67]. In japan, transplantation of a ABO incompatible kidney from a living donor is preferred to a deceased donor graft but the experience already acquired was extended in many other countries for recipients having only a ABO incompatible donor willing to donate [68].

The procedure involves a pretransplant treatment in order to remove the ABO antibody and to prevent furture production. Thus, Rrituximab is administred one month before transplan-tation followed by plasmapheresis 7 to 14 days before transplantation. With Rituximab there is no need for splenectomy and plasmapheresis is done in alternate days or even daily in order to reduce the ABO antibody titer under 8. The plasma removed is replaced with albumin solution and a combination of albumin and fresh frozen solution just immediately before transplantation to correct the coagulation. A key point is the administration of IVIG immediately after each plasmapheresis. The plasmapheresis is continued in the first two weeks after transplantation if ABO antibody titer was over 256 before Rituximab, if there is an increase of ABO antibody more than three times after transplantation, and if the serum creatinine increases more than 15% in two weeks after transplantation. The immunosuppression includes Tacrolimus, mycophenolate mofetil and steroids. In the first three weeks, the patient is at high risk of developing hyperacute humoral rejection, thus a graft biopsy is warranted whenever the serum creatinine increase over 15% in two weeks [69].

The use of specific immunoadsorbtion instead of plasmapheresis is not only less aggressive but also more effective since it allows more than two plasma exchange equivalent per one session [70].

Even if renal transplantation agains ABO blood group is expensive and, due to the increased immunosuppression, increases the infectious and malignancy risk, graft function at five years is slightly similar to transplantation of ABO compatible grafts [68].

2.9. Commercial renal transplantation

World Health Organization condemned the sales of organs since 1989. Sales of organs and tissues has been made illegal in the majority civilized states of the world. The difference between altruistic donation of a kidney and selling off a kidney is viewed as similar to the difference between marriage and prostitution. The first is a sacrament, the second a sin.

Reimbursement for expenses related to the donation process, such as for traveling and lodging is not prohibited, although a formal mechanism to make such reimbursements is not available everywhere, a factor that could act as a decentive to donation for some potential donors.

Iran is currently the only country in which payed donation is officially sanctioned, almost all the donors are pour and uneducated and follow-up studies have shown that their lives are not improved.

Despite the legal constraints on organ sales, commercial kidney transplantation is a common phenomena in many parts of the world, and in some cases has been linked to criminal activity. The donors are typical pour or under great financial stress, the recipients are often wealthy or come from other wealthier countries, and middleman or brokers are often involved.

Arguments against payed donation shows:

- The donor's choice is not voluntary because he is compelled by circumstances of poverty to donate a kidney. Poverty-stricken donors choose what they see as the best of a group of bed options. Compared to some other possibilities such working under unsafe conditions, kidney donation might carry less risk to the donor than other choices and at the same time might accomplish more good for society and for the donor.

- Paid donors are usually pour and uneducated, so making them understand the risks is all but impossible.

- Commercial donation will result in the rich having access to organs for transplantation while the pour do not.

- Donors will be exploited by unscrupulous middleman and sometimes, even by the surgeons. The medical care of both donor and recipient will suffer generally.

- The pour don't know how to handle the money that comes to them and will make no permanent difference in their poverty. This perception may be based on experience with lottery winners and other recipients of a sudden winfall. Donors will have widely differing abilities to plan for the future and would be difficult to predict what they will do with the payment for their donation. The possibility off misuse of money does not justify the overriding the donors wish to give up a kidney.

- During its entire history, transplantation has relayed on the altruism of donors and their families. Commercial donation would change the fundamental character of organ donation and likely would lead to the disappearance of altruistic donor. If any transplants are payed for, all will have to be. Most of payed donors are giving an organ to a specific individual. Payed donors would not have a choice about recipient. Thus, altruistic donation should continue.

- The initial enthusiastic support of organ transplantation has been replaced by suspicion. Although no evidence has proved the charges that are widely accepted urban myths regarding transplantation. This includes stories of people, particularly south-american children being kidnapped and killed for their organs, and people being drugged and kidnaped only to awaken in an alley with a flank incision and no kidney on that side. The myths can only be dispelled by the education, nothing else. Moreover, the possibility exists that skillful paper editors and television producers will exploit current practices for purposes of sensationalism.

Available data on the outcome of organ vending for the donors, indicates that the most of them have a pour outcome. On the other side, recipient of vended organ are subject to an increased risk for complications, particularly infections, likely as a result of a break-down of trust and honesty that is a byproduct of commercialization of organ donation. Evidence from several countries has shown that commercialization of organ donation comes at the expense of program for the related and unpaid living unrelated donation.

3. Cadaveric donation

The modest increase in cadaveric renal transplant in USA has been achieved in principally by extending use of older and younger donors [71]. Fortunately, the death from motor vehicle accidents has decreased over the passed 20 years mainly due to laws meant to increase the safety on the road: the seat belt laws, passive restraints, child safety seats, and stricter drunk driving laws. The greatest number of lives saved by improved highway safety has been specially at the 15 to 40 years old age group. On the other hand, another concern is related to the estimation that 10% of potential donors might be ineligible because of HIV infection [72].

In the same time, the number of older cadaver donors doubled between 1990 and 2000 especially due to a 10 fold increase in donors older than 60 years.

The percentage of donors dying in motor vehicle accidents decreased from 34.4% to 24.00% while the percentage of donors dying from stroke increased from 27% to 42% [71]. Despite the decrease in motor vehicle accidents, enough deaths still occur under circumstances that allow transplantation and could reduce the gap between the need for and the supply of kidneys in all civilized states in the world. The failure to make use of these organs has been attributed to the failure of the intensive care unit staff to recognize potential donors as well as the high refusal rate by families of potential cadaveric donors. Multiple new mechanisms for preventing potential donor from being missed in ICU appear to have been successful. Hospital staff are recognizing over two thirds of potential donors, are asking their families about donation but only half of them agree to donate.

Much attention has been focused on disparity among different ethnic groups as organ donors. A study of 1772 requested donation in come important cities from USA reported a family refusal rate of 17% in whites, 43% in Hispanics, and 45% in blacks [73], but the situation has changed in last period due to intensive efforts done to encourage minority families to donate. As a consequence the rate of cadaver kidney donation became similar for whites, blacks and Hispanics but remained low for Asians. Estimate of the overall refusal rate in the USA is between 38% to 50%. The refusal to donate lead to a 4755 kidneys lost for donation but the true potential in higher since we can't determine the real number of potential donors. This number would have enclosed 81% of the gap between the yearly increase in need and the available kidneys. Even so, the shortage of kidneys can not be closed by eligible donors lost by families refusal to donate and the difference would have to be provided by new cadaveric sources and by living donation.

3.1. Disparity among attitudes regarding cadaver donation

Even it might be only a believing, there is a dichotomy between the public and the medical community regarding cadaveric organ donation. The medical community is preferring cadaver organ donation since there are less concerns on the quality and risks associated with the donor's organs. Physicians don't share the cultural and religious believes of families opposed to organ donation. The doctors are relieved of concerns regarding doing harm to the donor because they often see the main problem as one that may be corrected by education and right information.

Even though over 90% of the public supports allowing living donation [74], many people do have reservations about cadaveric organ donation due to cultural and religious beliefs or beliefs that the dead can still suffer. The concept of brain death remains only a concept when it is about a loved one who has died unexpectedly. Families also express concern that the deceased's own wishes cannot be known or carried out. People might fear that being identified ahead of time as an organ donor would lead the medical team to make less than the maximal effort to save them [75].

3.2. Legislation means

An array of various laws have been passed to maximize the number of cadaveric donor transplants. In USA, the Uniform Anatomical Gift Act, have been passed for over 30 years by american Congress and authorize individuals to give their organs and specified who could give consent if the donor were unable to do so [76]. By now, many states have such a law in place and many of them use the driver license as a donor card.

"Routine inquiry" is active in many hospitals in Europe and USA. Majority of the hospitals who are doing or not transplantation, have routine inquiry policies which qualifies for social reimbursement. Hospitals are required to notify families of potential donors about the possibility of donation and to notify organ procurement agency approved by health care finance administration. In the first years after the passage of required request laws, donation increased slightly but then reached a new plateau.

Another way to approach organ donation, especially in European countries is that of presumed consent. Unless the potential donor has previously expressed a wish not to donate, he is presumed to have agreed to donate. The role of the family is to confirm that the deceased has not expressed an unwillingness to be a donor. The application of the law is variable and approximatively one half of the nations continues to depend on family consent in practice. The effect of donation have been variable; the refusal rate in Austria and Belgium, where the law is strictly applied dropped under 10%. In USA, public opinion shows little support for presumed consent law with only 7% supporting this approach.

An alternative to presumed consent has been proposed in the USA which is mandated choice [77]. When getting or renewing a driving license, a person would have to decide whether to become a potential donor, and the person's choice would take precedence over the family's wishes.

Another law which is active in some states in USA and some countries in Europe, is to provide a compensation for the donor's family. The fund for such thing is obtained by voluntary donations. One thing which is important here that the law makes the distinction between purchasing organs and bestowing a gift to the family in appreciation of its generosity.

3.3. Expanding donation criteria

When efforts that increase the consent rate for cadaver donors, another approach expanding the criteria for an acceptable cadaver donors, also has attempted to increase the number of kidneys available for transplantation. Less than 25% of the increase in cadaveric donors has come from traditional pool age 16 to 50 year age donors. The criteria have been expanded further in some instances by use of donors with encephalitis and core antibody positivity for hepatitis B [78]. Recent data have confirmed that safety of even using kidney from infected donors with blood cultures with pseudomonas and candida, provide appropriate antibiotic treatment is given [79]. There are studies which determined that bacteriemia accounted for 30% of medically unsuitable kidneys in brain death potential donor. There are also transplantation of horse shoe kidney [80] or kidneys from non renal organ transplant recipient which have to be mentioned. From any point you are going to look at this problem, the greatest potential to increase the potential donor pool comprises non-hard beating cadaver kidneys and kidneys from older donor.

Situations requiring edge biopsy
All people with normal renal function regardless of age (graft biopsy in donors over 60 years)
Diabetic donors with normal renal function and without severe proteinuria
All hypertensive donors with normal renal function
All hypotensive donors
Infected donors excluding viral hepatitis, HIV, Jakob-Creutzfeldt disease, viral encephalitis, malaria, disseminated TB
CMV + RPR
Positive urine cultures without pyelonephritis
Bacteremic donors
Donors with abnormal renal function
Donors at high risk for infection (but negative on high sensitive tests)
Donors with a history of malignancy disease-free for two years
Skin tumors without metastases, excluding melanoma
Primary CNS tumors without VP shunt

Adapted from [65]

Table 5. Expanded criteria for cadaveric donors

Non heart beating donors where widely used before the definition of brain death was accepted. They remain the major source of cadaver donors in countries such as Japan and Mexico, where brain death was recognized officially only recently and where social acceptance it is still limited [82]. Non heart beating donors yield about 5% of all cadaveric kidneys transplanted in USA. Use of non-heart beating cadaver donor kidneys has increased in last years. The one year survival of graft from non-heart beating donors was 83% and for brain death donors was 86%. Early function was not as good: 48% of recipient of non-heart beating donor kidneys required dialysis in the first week after transplantation compared to 22% of the recipients of kidneys from brain death donors. Primary non-function was slightly increased also (4% versus 1%). The serum creatinine level at discharge from hospital was higher in the first group. At one year follow-up, the serum creatinine levels for the two groups was, in fact, similar (1.9 mg/dL versus 1.8 mg/dL). When traumatic death were analyzed separately, the one year survival of non heart beating donors kidneys was 89% compared with 70% one year survival for non-traumatic death. Not all programs have found the same results from non-heart beating donors, but the finding of more frequent delayed function and need for dialysis has been universal. The potential for increasing the donor supply from non-heart beating donors has been estimated to be as high as 40% [83].

3.3.1. Older donors

Already, older donors are a major source of cadaveric donation. Some doctors found out an inferior outcome from transplants from cadaveric donors over 55 years of age. Not only did a higher percentage of recipients of such kidneys required dialysis but one year serum creatinine level was higher than that from recipient of transplants from cadaveric donors aged 5 to 55 years and the estimated halve life of the kidney was 5.8 +/- 0.3 years compared to 11+/- 0.3 years. Other analysis have found similar results but suggests that the adverse effects of the donor ages affect only certain subgroups particularly black recipients.

3.3.2. Hypertension

Recipients of kidneys from donors with hypertension were more likely to have anuria and to require dialysis immediately after transplantation. Their serum creatinine level was significant higher at one year than that of recipients of kidneys from donors who were not hypertensive and the predictive graft survival was shorter (halve life of 7.7 +/- 0.5 years versus 10.7 +/- 0.3 years). Graft survival was better with 1 to 5 years of hypertension compared to 6 or more years of hypertension. The difference in serum creatinine and predicted graft survival between kidneys from diabetic and non-diabetic donors was of borderline statistical significance. Serum creatinine at one year was 1.8 +/- 0.8 mg/dL in recipient of kidneys from diabetic donors compared with 1.6 +/- 0.8 mg/dL in recipients of kidney from non-diabetic donors. Predicted halve life in this graft was 8.4 +/- 1.5 years compared with 10.1 +/- 0.3 years.

3.4. Strategies for increasing organ donation

In developing new strategies for increasing kidney available for transplantation we would do well to remember that from its beginning organ transplantation has relied on public good will and support. When public opposition exists, we sometimes avoid using approaches that we find ethically acceptable. Because we really don't know what ideas or practices will strengthen public support for all organ donation the introduction of new practices should be undertaken as pilot projects.

The public already accept living donors who were not considered 50 years ago such unrelated living donors and spouses, which are now widely excepted. Once we accept the donors autonomy and remind ourselves that the risk to the donor is not related to his relationship to the recipient, we will be able to accept the wide arrange and greater number of emotionally related donors. We need to understand that the altruistic donor, although unusual, is not pathologic. The altruistic donor can be considered an emotionally related donor who is emotionally related to all mankind. Thus, this approach to this type of donor is not to keep a registry of willing donors and their HLA types. The altruistic donor is not waiting for the right HLA type but for the right story. The acceptance of donor autonomy would allow for accepting donors with increased risk, but will require careful follow-up thus an increased risk of complications can be recognized.

3.5. Conclusions

During the last period of time, there was a spite of papers from individual countries and registries, which examined the ways in which the number of kidney donors could be increased.

Most studies examined single initiatives, such as changing the transplant law, rather than the development of integrated donor programs. The act of donation is a complex phenomenon depending on many factors and interactions, few of which individually have been proven useful or generally applicable throw the out the european community. Well designed studies are needed urgently. A donation is the result of a chain of events, the final result of which will depend upon its weakest link.

Even when the individual links have been strengthened, each element of the process of donation must be integrated into the operational policies developed in toon with national moral and cultural values. It is easy to set a minimum standard to which countries should aspire. But it is another matter to recommend specific, donor promoting activities for which individual countries and profesional organizational should aim.

Although, living donor rate are no increasing in Europe, rates could be further improved at different stages in the referral process:

- Nephrologist at non transplanting as well as transplanting centers, should be encouraged to discuss openly the subject of living donation with family of patients suffering ESRD, preferably before the patient begins dialysis. This will results in predialysis transplantation, increased transplant rates, and is more efficient in case of reduced dialysis resources.

- Canceling facilities (e.g. by a senior nurse or living donor coordinators) should be available to discuss screening tests, provide information, and arrange eventually reimbursement of donor expenses allowed in law.

- Each transplant center should work to an approved screening protocol, such that the predicted mortality risk of living donation does not exceed 1 in 3000 cases.

- If legally permitted, living unrelated donors should be encouraged. In many countries in Europe, altruistic non related kidney donation is allowed legally, provided that checks are made for altruistic motivation and exclusion as far as possible of the possibility of organ sale.

- Non-directed living donor transplantation between altruistic donor and recipient unknown to the donor is possible and have been developed in few centers. Although controversial, there seem no moral or social reason to exclude such donors. However, there are ethical and legal concerns about this type of donation, which at the moment make it difficult to include in a recommendation list.

Increase supply and use of cadaveric kidneys:

Donor cards. In many countries publicity schemes encourage the population to carry donor cards, or to register their wish to donate (opting-in) on a computerized donor register. Even if in UK 8 mil. of individuals are now registered in the opting-in computer, only 10% of the population is currently caring donor cards. No more than 50 donor per year results from this initiative. For the success of such schemes, continuous publicity is essential to increase opted-in donors and transplant centers. Intensive care physicians and transplant coordinators should be mandated to access registry routinely, to identify the wishes of potential cadaveric donors.

Improved organization and resources. Services must be more organized and better resourced to increase cadaver donation. In several countries, the number of intensive care beds is probably too low to achieve more than 20 donors per million from intensive care patients. In high donating countries, with better resourced intensive care units, the staff responsible for donation (transplant coordinators), have been expanded and given proper financial support. Transplant coordinators are also to be given the responsibility of public relations, with the aim of avoiding adverse media publicity, and liaising with the coroners.

Opting-out legislation. The introduction of opting-out legislation appears on first site of the data available to be associated with the increased rates of cadaveric donation. In Europe, four countries which exceeded 20 kidneys donor per million population per annum, all have opting-out legislation. In France however, opting-out legislation has not achieved such a successful donation rates. This may be because France choose initially, hard line opting-out, in which donation takes place if the donor has not opted-out irrespective of families wishes. Adverse publicity led to a softening of the practice, which consequently increases the donation rates. Other countries which presumed consent law practices soft presumed consent, in which the families are taking into account in all situations. In general, countries with informed consent do not perform as well, main exception being USA, where kidney donation rates exceed 25 donors per million population.

Criteria for donor suitability. Non-heart beating donors (NHBD) are well known to produce a high rate of primary non-function and their acceptability was low. Recently introduced in situ perfusion of the dead bodies, which has been successfully developed in UK and Holland, are bringing in encouraging results. After harvesting, kidneys may be put into continuous perfusion machine, and their viability assessed using flow measurements and urinary and enzyme excretion. As a matter of fact, presumed consent legislation will allow more NHBD. Rapid intraarterial cold perfusion over recently deceased persons should be allowed before family consent low operate but perfusion without relatives permission is technically unwarranted assault. Agreement by a coroner should allow perfusion without permission and that could expand significantly NHBD.

Elderly donors. Even if long term survival for kidneys from elderly donors (over 60 years old) is 10-15% less than those taken from younger donors, better results may be obtained with carefully selected older donors and shortening of the cold ischemic time.

A good quality organ must be guaranteed to the recipient and every transplant center must established its own guidelines on organ acceptability. If the transplant center uses a less than optimum organs from old subjects to expand the pool of donors, the donors must be evaluated according to age, vascular condition and renal function. The inferior limit for a single kidney transplant is considered creatinine clearance more than 60 mL/min. If the calculated creatinine clearance is between 60 and 50 mL/min. the donor may be considered marginal. If the calculated creatinine clearance is less than 50 mL/min. than the kidney should not be used for a single transplantation, however, as they are organs that nobody wants they can be used for dual transplantation. When this policy is established, it is necessary to inform the patient on the waiting list.

Author details

Lucan Mihai*, Lucan Valerian Ciprian and Iacob Gheorghiță

*Address all correspondence to: mihai.lucan@gmail.com

Clinical Institute of Urology and Renal Transplantation, Cluj-Napoca, Romania

References

[1] Mandal AK, Kalligonis AN, Ratner LE. Expanded criteria donors: attempts to increase the renal transplant donor pool. Adv Ren Replace Ther. 2000;7(2):117-30.

[2] McBride MA, Harper AM, Taranto SE., The OPTN waiting list, 1988-2002. Clin Transpl. 2003:53-64.

[3] Walton-Moss BJ, Taylor L, Nolan MT. Ethical analysis of living organ donation. Prog Transplant. 2005;15(3):303-9.

[4] Lledó-Garcia E, Subirá-Ríos D, Tejedor-Jorge A, del Cañizo-López JF, Hernández-Fernández C. Optimizing outcomes by preconditioning the donor. Transplant Proc. 2011;43(1):349-52.

[5] Brar A, Jindal RM, Abbott KC, Hurst FP, Salifu MO. Practice patterns in evaluation of living kidney donors in United network for organ sharing-approved kidney transplant centers. Am J Nephrol. 2012;35(5):466-73.

[6] Goldfarb DA, Matin SF, Braun WE, Schreiber MJ, Mastroianni B, Papajcik D, Rolin HA, Flechner S, Goormastic M, Novick AC. Renal outcome 25 years after donor nephrectomy. J Urol. 2001;166(6):2043-7.

[7] Hung CJ, Lin YJ, Chang SS, Chou TC, Lee PC. Kidney grafts with multiple renal arteries is no longer a relative contraindication with advance in surgical techniques of laparoscopic donor nephrectomy. Transplant Proc. 2012;44(1):36-8.

[8] Tyson MD, Castle EP, Ko EY, Andrews PE, Heilman RL, Mekeel KL, Moss AA, Mulligan DC, Reddy KS. Living donor kidney transplantation with multiple renal arteries in the laparoscopic era. Urology. 2011;77(5):1116-21.

[9] Modlin CS, Goldfarb DA, Novick AC. The use of expanded criteria cadaver and live donor kidneys for transplantation. Urol Clin North Am. 2001;28(4):687-707.

[10] Lucan M., Tratat de tehnici chirurgicale urologice, ed. Infomedica, Bucuresti, 2001, p513-527.

[11] Nanidis TG, Antcliffe D, Kokkinos C, Borysiewicz CA, Darzi AW, Tekkis PP, Papalois VE. Laparoscopic versus open live donor nephrectomy in renal transplantation: a meta-analysis. Ann Surg. 2008;247(1):58-70.

[12] Dols LF, Kok NF, Ijzermans JN. Live donor nephrectomy: a review of evidence for surgical techniques. Transpl Int. 2010;23(2):121-30.

[13] Giessing M. Laparoscopic living-donor nephrectomy. Nephrol Dial Transplant. 2004;19 Suppl 4:iv36-40.

[14] Tooher RL, Rao MM, Scott DF, Wall DR, Francis DM, Bridgewater FH, Maddern GJ. A systematic review of laparoscopic live-donor nephrectomy. Transplantation. 200415;78(3):404-14.

[15] Moreira P, Sá H, Figueiredo A, Mota A. Delayed renal graft function: risk factors and impact on the outcome of transplantation. Transplant Proc. 2011;43(1):100-5.

[16] Bay WH, Hebert LA. The living donor in kidney transplantation. Ann Intern Med. 1987;106(5):719-27.

[17] Najarian JS, Chavers BM, McHugh LE, Matas AJ. 20 years or more of follow-up of living kidney donors. Lancet. 1992 3;340(8823):807-10.

[18] Fellner CH, Marshall JR. Kidney donors--the myth of informed consent. Am J Psychiatry. 1970;126(9):1245-51.

[19] Frade IC, Fonseca I, Dias L, Henriques AC, Martins LS, Santos J, Sarmento M, Lopes A. Impact assessment in living kidney donation: psychosocial aspects in the donor. Transplant Proc. 2008;40(3):677-81.

[20] Terasaki PI. The HLA-matching effect in different cohorts of kidney transplant recipients. Clin Transpl. 2000:497-514.

[21] 2001 Annual report. Vol. 1. Richmond, Va.: United Network for Organ Sharing, 2002:32.

[22] Abecassis M, Adams M, Adams P, et all; Live Organ Donor Consensus Group. Consensus statement on the live organ donor. JAMA. 2000;284(22):2919-26.

[23] Scheper-Hughes N. Keeping an eye on the global traffic in human organs. Lancet. 2003;361(9369):1645-8.

[24] Cohen L. Where it hurts: Indian material for an ethics of organ transplantation. Daedalus. 1999;128(4):135-65.

[25] Siminoff LA, Chillag K. The fallacy of the "gift of life". Hastings Cent Rep. 1999;29(6): 34-41.

[26] Green RM: What does it mean to use someone as "a means only": rereading Kant. Kennedy Inst Ethics J 2001, 11(3):247-61

[27] Campbell CS: Body, Self, and the property paradigm. Hastings Cent Rep 1992, 22(5): 34-42

[28] Boulware LE, Troll MU, Wang NY, Powe NR. Public attitudes toward incentives for organ donation: a national study of different racial/ethnic and income groups. Am J Transplant. 2006 Nov;6(11):2774-85

[29] Goyal M, Mehta RL, Schneiderman LJ, Sehgal AR. Economic and health consequences of selling a kidney in India. JAMA 2002; 288:1589-1593

[30] National Organ Transplant Act: Public Law 98-507. US Statut Large 1984; 98

[31] Israni AK, Halpern SD, Zink S, Sidhwani SA, Caplan A. Incentive models to increase living kidney donation: Encouraging without coercing. Am J Transplant 2005; 5: 15–20

[32] William Frist, S. 2283 (109th): Gift of Life Congressional Medal Act of 2006, 109th Congress, 2005–2006.

[33] Fortney Stark, H.R. 4753 (109th): Gift of Life Congressional Medal Act of 2006,109th Congress, 2005–2006.

[34] Ross LF, Woodle ES. Ethical issues in increasing living kidney donations by expanding kidney paired exchange programs. Transplantation. 2000;69(8):1539-43.

[35] Smith C. She saves mom, gets fired for it. Seattle Post-Intellinger. November 22, 2001.].

[36] Public law No. 106-56, Organ donor leave act, H.R. 457, USA Congress

[37] Office of the Assistant Secretary for Planning and Evaluation, Depart-ment of Health and Human Services. Standards for Privacy of Individually Identifiable Health Information: Final rule. Fed Regist 2000;65(250): 82475, 82803-5, 82810, 82812-3.

[38] Ellison MD, McBride MA, Taranto SE, Delmonico FL, Kauffman HM. Living kidney donors in need of kidney transplants: a report from the organ procurement and transplantation network. Transplantation. 2002;74(9):1349-51.

[39] Matas AJ, Bartlett ST, Leichtman AB, Delmonico FL. Morbidity and mortality after living kidney donation, 1999-2001: survey of United States transplant centers. Am J Transplant. 2003;3(7):830-4.

[40] Wallis CB, Samy KP, Roth AE, Rees MA. Kidney paired donation. Nephrol Dial Transplant. 2011 Jul;26(7):2091-9

[41] Montgomery RA, Cooper M, Kraus E et al. Renal transplantation at the Johns Hopkins Comprehensive Transplant Center. Clin Transpl 2003: 199–213

[42] Gentry SE, Segev DL, Simmerling M et al. Expanding kidney paired donation through participation by compatible pairs. Am J Transplant 2007; 7: 2361–2370

[43] de Klerk M, Keizer KM, Claas FH et al. The Dutch national living donor kidney exchange program. Am J Transplant 2005; 5: 2302–2305

[44] Montgomery RA. Renal transplantation across HLA and ABO antibody barriers: integrating paired donation into desensitization protocols. Am J Transplant 2010; 10: 449–457

[45] Delmonico FL, Morrissey PE, Lipkowitz GS et al. Donor kidney exchanges. Am J Transplant 2004; 4: 1628–1634

[46] Roth AE, Sonmez T, Unver MU, Delmonico FL, Saidman SL. Util- izing list exchange and nondirected donation through 'chain' paired kidney donations. Am J Transplant 2006; 6: 2694–2705

[47] Gentry SE, Segev DL, Montgomery RA. A comparison of populations served by kidney paired donation and list paired donation. Am J Transplant 2005; 5: 1914–1921

[48] den Hartogh G. Trading with the waiting-list: the justice of living donor list exchange. Bioethics 2010; 24: 190–198

[49] Gilbert JC, Brigham L, Batty DS Jr. et al. The nondirected living donor program: a model for cooperative donation, recovery and allocation of living donor kidneys. Am J Transplant 2005; 5: 167–174

[50] Cecka JM. The UNOS Scientific Renal Transplant Registry--2000. Clin Transpl. 2000:1-18.

[51] Eggers P. Comparison of treatment costs between dialysis and transplantation. Semin Nephrol. 1992;12(3):284-9.

[52] O'Connor KJ, Delmonico FL. Increasing the supply of kidneys for transplantation. Semin Dial. 2005;18(6):460-2.

[53] Fehrman-Ekholm I. Living donor kidney transplantation. Transplant Proc. 2006;38(8):2637-41.

[54] Clayman RV, Kavoussi LR, Soper NJ, Dierks SM, Meretyk S, Darcy MD, Roemer FD, Pingleton ED, Thomson PG, Long SR. Laparoscopic nephrectomy: initial case report. J Urol. 1991;146(2):278-82.

[55] Kerbl K, Clayman RV, McDougall EM, Gill IS, Wilson BS, Chandhoke PS, Albala DM, Kavoussi LR. Transperitoneal nephrectomy for benign disease of the kidney: a comparison of laparoscopic and open surgical techniques. Urology. 1994;43(5): 607-13.

[56] Kavoussi LR, Kerbl K, Capelouto CC, McDougall EM, Clayman RV. Laparoscopic nephrectomy for renal neoplasms. Urology. 1993;42(5):603-9.

[57] Rassweiler J, Fornara P, Weber M, Janetschek G, Fahlenkamp D, Henkel T, Beer M, Stackl W, Boeckmann W, Recker F, Lampel A, Fischer C, Humke U, Miller K. Laparoscopic nephrectomy: the experience of the laparoscopy working group of the German Urologic Association. J Urol. 1998;160(1):18-21.

[58] Benoit G, Blanchet P, Moukarzel M, Hiesse C, Bensadoun H, Bellamy J, Charpentier B, Jardin A. Surgical complications in kidney transplantation. Transplant Proc. 1994;26(1):287-8.

[59] Brown SL, Biehl TR, Rawlins MC, Hefty TR. Laparoscopic live donor nephrectomy: a comparison with the conventional open approach. J Urol. 2001;165(3):766-9.

[60] Levey AS, Danovitch G, Hou S. Living donor kidney transplantation in the United States--looking back, looking forward. Am J Kidney Dis. 2011;58(3):343-8.

[61] Davis CL, Delmonico FL. Living-donor kidney transplantation: a review of the current practices for the live donor. J Am Soc Nephrol. 2005;16(7):2098-110.

[62] Ratner LE, Montgomery RA, Kavoussi LR. Laparoscopic live donor nephrectomy. A review of the first 5 years. Urol Clin North Am. 2001;28(4):709-19.

[63] Montgomery RA, Lonze BE, King KE, Kraus ES, Kucirka LM, Locke JE, Warren DS, Simpkins CE, Dagher NN, Singer AL, Zachary AA, Segev DL. Desensitization in HLA-incompatible kidney recipients and survival. N Engl J Med. 2011;365(4):318-26.

[64] Rapaport FT. The case for living emotionally related international kidney donor exchange registry. Transplant Proc 1986; 18(suppl 2): 5-9.

[65] Gentry S, Segev DL. Living donor kidney exchange. Clin Transpl. 2011:279-86.

[66] Lucan M. Five years of single-center experience with paired kidney exchange transplantation. Transplant Proc. 2007;39(5):1371-5.

[67] Tanabe K, Takahashi K, Sonda K, Tokumoto T, Ishikawa N, Kawai T, et al. Long-term results of ABO-incompatible living kidney transplantation: a single-center experience. Transplantation 1998;65:224-8

[68] Crew RJ, Ratner LE. ABO-incompatible kidney transplantation: current practice and the decade ahead. Curr Opin Organ Transplant. 2010;15(4):526-30.].

[69] Jeon BJ, Kim IG, Seong YK, Han BH. Analysis of the Results of ABO-Incompatible Kidney Transplantation: In Comparison with ABO-Compatible Kidney Transplantation. Korean J Urol. 2010;51(12):863-9.

[70] Genberg H, Kumlien G, Wennberg L, Tyden G. The efficacy of antigen-specific immunoadsorption and rebound of anti-A/B antibodies in ABO-incompatible kidney transplantation. Nephrol Dial Transplant. 2011;26(7):2394-400.

[71] 1998 Annual Report. U.S. Scientific Registry of Transplant Recipients and the Organ Procurement and Transplantation Network. Transplant Data 1988–1997. Richmond, U.S. Department of Health and Human Services, Office of Special Programs, Division of Transplantation, UNOS

[72] Evans RW, Orians CE, Ascher NL. The potential supply of organ donors. JAMA 1992, 267:239–246

[73] Perez LM, Schulman B, Davis F, Olson L, Tellis VA, Matas AJ. Organ donation in three large American cities with large Latino and black populations. Transplantation 1998, 46:553–557

[74] Spital A, Spital M. Living kidney donation: Attitudes outside the transplant center. Arch Intern Med 1988, 148:1077–1080

[75] Callender CO, Hall LE, Yeager CL, Barber JB, Dunston GM, Pinn-Wiggins VW. Organ donation and blacks: A critical frontier. N Engl J Med 1991, 325:442–444

[76] Stuart FP, Veith FJ, Cranford RE. Braindeath laws and patterns of consent to remove organs for transplantation from cadavers in the United States and 28 other countries. Transplantation 1981, 31:238–244

[77] Spital A. Mandated choice for organ donation: Time to give it a try. Ann Intern Med 1996, 125:66–69

[78] Madayag RM, Johnson LB, Bartlett ST, Schweitzer EJ, Constantine NT, McCarter RJ, Kuo PC, Keay S, Oldach DW. Use of renal allografts from donors positive for hepatitis B core antibody confers minimal risk for subsequent development of clinical hepatitis B virus disease. Transplantation 1967; 64:1781–1786

[79] Freeman RB, Giatras I, Falagas ME, Supran S, O'Conner K, Bradley J, Snydman DR, Delmonico FL. Outcome of transplantation of organs procured from bacteremic donors. Transplantation 1999; 68:1107–1111

[80] Thomson BNJ, Francis DM, Millar RJ. Transplantation of adult and paediatric horseshoe kidneys. Aust NZJ Surg 1997; 67:279–282

[81] Alexander JW. Expanded Donor Criteria: Background and Suggestions for Kidney Donation. Richmond, Report of the UNOS Ad Hoc Donations Committee, 1991

[82] Hiraga S, Kitamura M, Kakuta T, Takebayashi Y, Fukuuchi F, Kitajima N, Hida M: Clinical outcome of cadaveric renaltransplantation with non-heart-beating donors: Special reference to serious complications. Transplant Proc 1997; 29:3561–3564

[83] ChoY W, Terasaki PI, Cecka JM, Gjertson DW. Transplantation of kidneys from donors whose hearts have stopped beating. N Engl J Med 1998; 338:221–225

Chapter 4

Overview of Immunosuppression in Renal Transplantation

M. Ghanta, J. Dreier, R. Jacob and I. Lee

Additional information is available at the end of the chapter

1. Introduction

The use of potent induction agents and maintenance immunosuppression has substantially decreased the risk of acute rejection. One year graft survival is greater than 92% in deceased donor and 96% in living donor transplant recipients with current immunosuppressive strategies according to the Scientific Registry of Transplant Recipients, (SRTR, 2009).

Half life appears to be the best way to give the patient a general understanding of how long their transplant may last. The graft half life for deceased donor transplants has increased from 6.6 years in 1989 to 8.8 years by 2005. Significant progress has also been made in high risk transplants where graft half life has improved from 3 years in 1989 to 6.4 years in 2005 for expanded criteria donor recipients. For the standard low risk patient receiving a living donor kidney, current immunosuppression should guarantee a graft half life of at least 11.9 years. [1]

However, the problems of chronic rejection and chronic allograft dysfunction still remain, often leading to graft loss and shortened long-term graft survival.[2] The 5 and 10 year adjusted graft survival for deceased donor transplants were 70% and 43% respectively. The adjusted 5 year and 10 year graft survival for living donor transplant were 82% and 60% respectively. (SRTR, 2009)

Humoral rejection and sensitized patients continue to be a clinical challenge. The management and clinical impact of subclinical rejection also remains unclear. Although there are numerous clinical trials testing different immunosuppressive strategies, a lack of large prospective randomized clinical trials has decreased our ability to generate consensus on the best immunosuppressive strategies for preserving long-term allograft function. This chapter will focus on reviewing multiple aspects of immunosuppressive therapy, such as; 1) mechanism of action, 2) how therapies are being utilized in practice, 3) the advantages and/or disadvantages of different therapies and 4) major clinical trials evaluating the effectiveness of specific regimens. New emerging strategies and therapeutic agents that are being investigated will also be discussed.

2. Induction agents

The goal of induction therapy is to suppress both cellular and humoral responses to prevent episodes of acute rejection. Rabbit anti-thymocyte globulin (rATG), IL-2 receptor blockers, and Alemtuzumab (Campath), are the primary antilymphocyte antibody preparations that are currently used for induction. More than 80% of the transplant centers in the United States use induction agents immediately post transplantation.[3] The specific agent utilized is often based on multiple factors which include recipient risk for rejection, recipient race, presence of chronic infections such as Hepatitis B or C, HIV, and center preference. See Table 1. for common induction agents.

2.1. Thymoglobulin

Thymoglobulin (rATG) is the most commonly used induction agent in United States. (rATG), is an antilymphocyte polyclonal antibody that is derived by injecting rabbits with human thymocytes. rATG contains polyclonal cytotoxic antibodies mainly targeted against various epitopes on human T lymphocytes and works primarily by complement mediated depletion of T lymphocytes. However, the multiple specificities of rATG against a broad range of T-cell antigens can affect multiple pathways involved in T-cell trafficking, adhesion, activation and promotion of certain T-cell subsets that may be more favorable for transplantation such as T-regulatory cells. [4-6] Although primarily a T-cell directed agent, the development of humoral responses which are dependent on T-cell help are likely compromised by rATG as well.

2.1.1. Side effects

Secondary to potential infusion reactions and other toxicities, administration of rATG requires patient monitoring and is administered in an inpatient setting or in an established infusion center. The typical dose is 1.5mg/kg/dose and involves 3-5 doses of rATG, depending on center protocols.

The antibodies in rATG can bind to proteins on the surface of granulocytes as well as platelets and hence leucopenia and thrombocytopenia are commonly encountered after rATG administration. Cytopenias are handled either by dose reduction or holding the dose. Despite premedication, infusion reactions do occur including fevers, chills and arthralgias. Serious reactions such as anaphylaxis, acute respiratory distress syndrome (noncardiogenic pulmonary edema) occur rarely. Typically these reactions are a result of intense cytokine release from lysis of T lymphocytes. Since rATG is obtained from rabbit sera, serum sickness can occur which presents with fever, malaise, diffuse arthralgias and rash. rATG results in prolonged T cell depletion, up to 6 months post administration and recipients are at increased risk for opportunistic infections and lymphoma. Patients are typically prophylaxed for cytomegalo-virus infection and pneumocystis carinii infection post rATG administration.

2.2. Alemtuzumab

Alemtuzumab or Campath is a recombinant humanized monoclonal antibody directed against CD52. It binds to CD52 receptor on the surface of T and B lymphocytes leading to antibody mediated cell lysis. CD52 is present on virtually all B and T cells as well as macrophages, NK cells and some granulocytes. It was initially approved for use in B-cell lymphocytic leukemia and is now used in transplantation. Alemtuzumab induces a rapid and profound depletion of peripheral and central lymphoid cells. It is typically administered as a single 30 mg dose either subcutaneously or intravenously. Just like rATG patients receive premedication to prevent infusion reactions. When used as an induction agent it is given intraoperatively. Single dose administration makes Campath a more convenient option to administer compared to rATG which is typically administered daily for 3-5 days.

2.2.1. Side effects

Potential side effects include thrombocytopenia, vomiting, diarrhea, headache and rarely auto-immune hemolytic anemia. Infection and lymphoma risk is similar to rATG, and patients are similarly prophylaxed for potential infections.

2.3. IL-2 receptor blockers (IL-2RA)

IL-2 receptor blockers, Basiliximab (Simulect) and daclizumab (Zenapax) are humanized anti-CD25 monoclonal antibody preparations. They are targeted against the α-chain (CD25) of the IL-2 receptor. Rather than working by lymphocyte depletion, these agents block IL-2 signaling which is required for T-cell growth, differentiation and expansion. Because both agents are derived from mice and partly humanized, they cause far less infusion reactions compared to rATG. Daclizumab is currently not available for use in United States. Basiliximab is used in the U.S. and is typically administered as 20mg intravenous infusion intraoperatively with subsequent doses given on the third or fourth post operative day. Neither drug has major side effects. Risk of infection and lymphoma is far less than that of lymphocyte depleting agents.

3. Which induction agent?

According to the annual report from SRTR 2009, 83% of transplant recipients received induction agents at the time of kidney transplant. The majority of patients received a T-cell depleting agent, 58%, and 21.2% received an IL-2 receptor blocking agent.

How agents are used in practice is dependent on a number of factors which range from center specific protocols to tailored immunosuppression based on recipient factors. The risks and benefits of each agent must be assessed in every patient individually based on the individuals' immunologic risk and susceptibility to infectious complications. Induction agents clearly possess different mechanisms of action that will have different effects on modulating cellular and humoral immune responses. It may be more advantageous to use more potent induction therapies such as the lymphocyte depleting agents, in those recipients at higher risk for rejection. On the other hand, utilizing such agents may be of concern in recipients with chronic infections such as hepatitis B and/or C or HIV. [7-10]

Induction Agents	Thymoglobulin
	Basiliximab
	Daclizumab
	Alemtuzumab
	Rituximab
Maintenance Agents	Tacrolimus
	Cyclosporine
	Sirolimus
	Mycofenolate Mofetil
	Azathioprine
	Corticosteroids
	Belatacept
	Leflunomide

Table 1. Immunosuppressive agents

Lymphocyte depleting agents such as rATG and Alemtuzumab primarily differ in their ability to deplete specific types of leukocytes. rATG contains polyclonal antibodies directed at thymic antigens and is more T-cell directed, and has little direct effect on B-cell depletion. Alemtuzumab contains a specific monoclonal antibody against CD52 which is expressed by both T and B cells as well as antigen presenting cells (APCs). The effect of Alemtuzumab mechanistically is directed at disabling several arms of the immune response, such as cell mediated (T-cell responses) and humorally mediated (B-cells) responses, as well as affecting antigen presenting cells.

Existing studies however, fail to show greater efficacy of Alemtuzumab compared to rATG in clinical trials. However, case series and other small trials speak of the benefit of utilizing Alemtuzumab in refractory rejection, and in instances of mixed rejection where an agent with activity against both cell mediated and humoral responses are required. Finally, both Alemtuzumab and rATG are agents of choice in patients that are considered higher risk such as African American race, repeat renal transplant, and sensitized patients with high panel reactivity to multiple HLA antigens.

The IL-2 receptor blocker, Basiliximab (Simulect), provides an option for induction therapy in those recipients with history of chronic infections with hepatitis B and or C and HIV, as Simulect is associated with less infectious complications post-transplant compared to lymphocyte depleting agents. Less immunosuppression is also an attractive option for those patients who may not require potent induction therapy, such as recipients that are older,

Caucasian, and those receiving living donor kidneys. When compared to lymphocyte depleting agents, clinical trials suggest more acute rejection episodes with IL-2RA. [11]

Utilizing data from the United Network For Organ Sharing Data Registry, a recent study
examining a large cohort of HIV recipients demonstrated higher risk of DGF and death
censored graft loss with IL-2 receptor agents.[12] HIV patients also have higher rates of
acute rejection with one recent study reporting a 31% incidence at one year.[7] Questions
remain as to whether this is driven in part by choosing a less potent induction agent
such as Simulect or issues with achieving therapeutic levels and/or avoiding toxic levels
of maintenance drugs that interact with many anti-retroviral HIV medications. Thymoglobulin has been used in HIV recipients but can lower the CD4+ cell count dramatically,
with recovery occurring as far out as two years. [13] Thymoglobulin use in HIV has also
been associated with increased risk of infections requiring hospitalizations. Clearly, more
studies are needed to weigh the risks and benefits of IL-2 receptor blockers on long-term
graft function and post-transplant infectious complications.

4. Comparison of induction agents; clinical trials

A study by Terasaki et al analyzed the various induction immunosuppression strategies used
across centers in the United States [3]. From 2003 onwards, the majority of centers were
utilizing Simulect, rATG or Alemtuzumab. According to the OPTN database, recipients who
received alemtuzumab had the lowest risk of graft failure, followed by rATG and basiliximab.
However, the benefit of one induction agent over the other is not entirely clear because
conclusions from small single center studies and retrospective studies utilizing database
reviews are often mixed. In addition, studies may be difficult to evaluate secondary to different
maintenance regimens that are used after induction.

Larger randomized trials and multicenter trials have been conducted and generally demonstrate that cell-depleting agents are generally more efficacious than IL2RA induction.
[3] In a randomized controlled trial, rATG was superior to IL2RA in preventing acute rejection in recipients with high-immunologic risk, and with standard criteria donor kidneys. Two prospective randomized trials demonstrated rATG was superior to basiliximab
in preventing biopsy proven acute rejection in standard criteria donor kidney recipients.
When comparing Alemtuzumab to rATG, studies are mixed. In a separate single center
randomized trial comparing alemtuzumab with rATG induction, Farney et al have
shown that alemtuzumab is superior to rATG in preventing biopsy proven acute rejection.[14] However, in a larger randomized multicenter study (INTAC), Hanaway et al
compared induction therapy with alemtuzumab to conventional induction (basiliximab or
rATG). At one year post transplant, the incidence of biopsy proven acute rejection was
lower in the alemtuzumab arm compared to basiliximab induction in low immunologic
risk recipients. However in the high immunologic risk recipients, alemtuzumab was as
efficacious but not superior to rATG.

5. Induction agents in sensitized patients

Rituximab (Rituxan) is used in the following clinical scenarios; 1) ABO incompatible or positive cross match transplantation, 2) treatment of antibody mediated rejection and 3) desensitization by decreasing titers of preformed alloantibodies prior to transplantation. [15-17] It is an anti-CD20 monoclonal antibody directed against the CD20 antigen present on naive B-cell lymphocytes. It creates a rapid and sustained depletion of circulating naive B cells for approximately 6 months. Because of its specific activity against B-cells, Rituxan is used to target the humoral arm of the immune response by limiting B-cell activity and antibody production. Although widely used in transplantation, the efficacy of this drug when compared with other newer agents in treating humoral responses and decreasing alloantibody production remains to be seen.

Eculizumab, is an anti C5 antibody which leads to terminal complement blockade and prevents formation of the membrane attack complex. Eculizumab protects allografts from complement mediated injury which occurs when pathogenic alloantibodies directed against donor allograft tissue activate complement. Although not widely used yet, the Mayo Clinic published an open label study demonstrating that blockade of terminal complement decreases antibody mediated rejection in sensitized patients and allows for positive crossmatch transplantation to occur. Eculizumab reduced antibody mediated rejection (AMR) to 7.7% compared to historical control groups where the incidence of AMR was 30-40% in the first few months.[18] Compared to long-standing protocols widely used for sensitized patients (e.g, plasmapharesis, IVIG and Rituximab), Eculizumab looks more promising in decreasing AMR rates.

Bortezomib, is a proteasome inhibitor that has specific activity against high affinity antibody producing plasma cells (PC), and induces apoptosis of circulating PC (a small percentage of the PC population) but in addition is able to effect PC that remain in survival niches such as the bone marrow and spleen.[19] Besides affecting the humoral arm, Bortezomib has multiple effects on immune cell function. Proteosome inhibition prevents the function of NFκB, an important transcription factor that transcribes multiple genes important for immune cell function and disrupts the regulation of cell cycle proteins, cell survival signals and expression of adhesion molecules.[20, 21] In transplantation it is used to treat refractory antibody mediated rejection as well as to reduce the burden of preformed alloantibodies to facilitate transplantation of highly sensitized individuals. Studies and case series evaluating the use of Bortezomib for desensitization and treatment of acute rejection have been mixed.[22-25] Although used by some centers, it has not been widely adopted into practice.

6. Maintenance immunosuppression

Maintenance therapy is used to prevent acute rejection and promote long term graft survival. Conventionally, combinations of 2-3 drugs with different mechanisms of action targeting various immune responses are used. Maintenance regimens vary according to the center, immunological risk of the patient, and individual susceptibility to adverse reactions. The introduction of calcineurin inhibitors (CNI) together with anti-proliferative agents like mycophenolate mofetil has resulted in major improvements in acute rejection rates and short term graft survival over the last three decades in kidney transplant recipients. However, long term graft outcomes have not improved dramatically, partly because of nephrotoxicities associated with the long term use of these drugs. In the year 2009, the initial maintenance regimen for 81% of kidney transplant recipients included tacrolimus and mycophenolate mofetil, per SRTR report, 2009. At one year post transplantation, 72.1% of the kidney transplant recipients remained on tacrolimus and mycophenolate moefetil and only 5.3% were receiving cyclosporine and mycophenolate mofetil. See Table 1 for common maintenance agents.

Although the majority of US centers utilize CNI in combination with mycophenolate moefetil for maintenance, different dosing strategies for CNI, as well as new agents are being explored. A recently FDA approved medication for use in renal transplant, Belatacept, may have a promising role in widescale maintenance immunosuppression in the future. The basic pharmacology, clinical uses, major drug interactions and toxicity profiles of commonly used and new maintenance agents will be discussed in this section.

6.1. Calcineurin inhibitors

Since their introduction in the 1970s, CNI have been the fundamental agents used for maintenance immunosuppression in solid organ transplantation. They played a revolutionary role in transplantation by dramatically reducing the incidence of acute rejection episodes and prolonging allograft survival post-transplant. Cyclosporine and tacrolimus are the available CNI preparations with both having a unique role in maintenance. Currently, tacrolimus is more widely used compared to cyclosporine primarily because there is less nephrotoxicity associated with tacrolimus. Based on recent SRTR reporting, the use of cyclosporine has declined from 66.3% in 1998 to 5.7% in 2009. Notably the use of tacrolimus has increased from 25.9% to 87.8%.

6.2. Mechanism of action of CNI

The target protein of both tacrolimus and cyclosporine is CNI which is a calcium-dependent phosphatase. This enzyme is ubiquitously expressed and associates with calmodulin to form an active enzyme complex that dephosphorylates and activates the transcription factor, nuclear factor of activated T cells (NFAT), after T-cell receptor signaling. Dephosphorylated NFAT can then translocate to the nucleus and initiate transcription of several key cytokine genes (e.g., IL-2, IL-4, TNF- and IFN-γ). Blockade of calcineurin leads to decreased NFAT activity and transcription of critical cytokines affecting T cell function, activation and proliferation. Both these drugs bind to cytoplasmic proteins to mediate their action. Cyclosporin binds to cyclophilin, while tacrolimus binds to FKBP-12.

6.3. Clinical use

Recommended starting dose for tacrolimus is 0.15-0.30 mg/kg, while that of cyclosporine is 6-10 mg/kg. For both drugs, total dose is administered in two divided doses. Intravenous dosing is 1/3rd of the total oral dose, administered as a continuous 24 hour infusion. Patient variability in drug kinetics can be attributed to the heterogeneity of metabolic activity of the enzyme responsible for calcineurin metabolism; the liver enzyme, CYP3A. In general, African Americans may require higher doses of tacrolimus, whereas patients with liver disease and elderly patients may need lower doses. Because of wide patient variability in metabolism, therapeutic drug monitoring is routinely performed with these agents. Most centers check a 12 hr trough level prior to the morning dose. More sophisticated monitoring with area under the curve (AUC) measurements is available but is not routinely performed because of technical and clinical difficulties. During the first 3 months post transplant, our center aims for a 12 hr tacrolimus trough in the range of 8-12 ng/dl, followed by a level of 6-10 ng/dl for months 4 to 12. After the first year, we reduce tacrolimus dosing aiming to achieve maintenance levels of of 4-6 ng/dl. For cyclosporine, a 12 hour trough of 250-350 mg/dl are maintained for the first few months and then target levels are gradually decreased. After the first year post transplantation the usual cyclosporine trough is between 100-200mg/dl. Targeted drug ranges vary across centers and are driven by center protocols that take into account patient risk, type of induction used and the strength of other agents used for maintenance.

6.4. Metabolism of CNIs and major drug interactions

Both tacrolimus and cyclosporine are metabolized by cytochrome P450 (CYP3a) enzymes that are located in the GI tract and liver. Both drugs are excreted in bile so dosage adjustment is not needed in renal insufficiency. Many medications are metabolized by P450 system and therefore many potential and significant drug interactions with CNI can occur. Classes of drugs that induce CYP3a can reduce CNI levels, such that increased dosing may be required to reach therapeutic and adequate ranges. On the other hand, drugs that block the action of CYP3a can lead to increased levels of CNI, which can lead to acute nephrotoxicity among other side effects. Specific blood pressure medications, antibiotics, anti-fungals, anti-convulsants and HIV medications need to be reviewed for p450 interactions, and both CNI and medications need to be adjusted accordingly. Commonly used medications that affect P450, and the subsequent impact on CNI levels are shown in Table 2.

Agents that are not often considered in practice, but having an effect on CNI include, steroids which when withdrawn can lead to increases in drug levels of CNIs, and binders such as cholestyramine and sevelamer which can bind CNIs and prevent absorption leading to sub therapeutic levels. Grape fruit juice increases absorption of tacrolimus and hence it is generally recommended to avoid its use with CNIs. Several herbal medications can also alter the metabolism of these drugs.

Because of the sensitive interactions between CNI and antiretrovirals, mangagement of CNI in HIV recipients can be challenging. CNI toxicity and supra therapeutic levels of CNI are common issues in HIV recipients and most likely contributes to allograft dyfunction. Reduced dosing of Tacrolimus is required with some protease inhibitors, particularly Ritonavir, the most potent blocker of CYP3A, and is dosed once to twice a week as opposed to the normal twice a day dosing.

Increases CNI level by inhibition of P450	Decreases CNI level by induction of P450
* Verapamil	Rifampin
Amlodipine	Rifabutin
* Diltiazem	Barbiturates
Nicardipine	Phenytoin
* Ketoconazole	Carbamazepine
Fluconazole	
Itraconazole	
Voriconazole	
Erythromycin	
Ritonavir	

*Significant increases in CNI level

Table 2. CNI-Drug Interactions

6.5. Adverse effects and toxicities of CNI

CNIs have facilitated the success of transplantation and a greater number of patients are living with functioning transplants for longer periods of time. This has made long term CNI exposure and the associated side effects inevitable. Cyclosporine and tacrolimus possess unique side effect profiles which play an important role in agent selection for individual patients.

One of the most significant side effects of CNIs is nephrotoxicity which contributes to chronic allograft dysfunction and late allograft loss. Acute CNI toxicity is functionally mediated by vasoconstriction of the afferent arteriole leading to reduction in renal blood flow and glomerular filtration rate. Studies demonstrate that CNI increases renin production in the kidney leading to angiotensin II mediated vasoconstriction. [26] Chronic exposure can lead to prolonged vasoconstriction and acute tubular necrosis. Chronic CNI nephrotoxicity can mediate vascular injury, glomerular ischemia, tubular atrophy and chronic interstitial fibrosis. Basic studies do demonstrate that excess production of fibrosing cytokines like transforming growth factor beta (TGF-β) is in part driven by CNI direct role on renin secretion in the kidney. [27] The development of calcineurin minimization and withdrawal protocols as well as the development of new maintenance agents are an attempt to prevent/minimize CNI nephrotoxicity and its impact on long-term allograft survival.

Other adverse renal manifestations of CNIs include thrombotic microangiopathy, which presents with renal dysfunction, microangiopathic hemolytic anemia and thrombocytopenia. CNI can also cause isolated tubular toxicity which manifests in many forms of electrolyte disturbances. The most prominent and clinically significant of these are renal tubular acidosis (RTA) type 4 (typically associated with metabolic acidosis and hyperkalemia) and hypomagnesemia. Proposed mechanisms mediating this effect includes, decreased aldosterone production secondary to cyclosporine, as well as decreased transcription and expression of mineralocorticoid receptor due to prograf.

Since calcineurin is a ubiquitous enzyme, there are other non-renal toxicities associated with CNI use. Tacrolimus is associated with neurotocity, GI side effects and pancreatic islet toxicity. Neurotoxicity can be as benign as tremors, but in some cases can be quite severe and lead to seizures and altered mental status. Finally, Tacrolimus use has been associated with posterior reversible encephalopathy syndrome (PRES) which can present with various neurological manifestations.[28] Another important clinical issue is the development of new onset post-transplant diabetes, or worsening diabetes post-transplant, particularly with tacrolimus. Neuro and pancreatic toxicity of tacrolimus are clinically handled by either dose reduction or conversion to cyclosporine. Cyclosporine use however can cause gingival hyperplasia, hirsutism, hypercholesterolemia, hypertension, salt retention and an increased incidence of gout. Both CNIs have been linked to increased risk of infectious complications as well as post transplant malignancies. Differences in adverse effects among the CNIs as well as other maintenance agents are shown in Table 3.

The current challenge is to mitigate the side effects of CNIs without sacrificing overall graft outcomes. Several novel protocols are recently designed and studied to overcome CNI toxicity. We have summarized these in the section of new evolving protocols.

6.6. Mycophenolate mofetil

Mycophenolate mofetil (MMF) is a maintenance immunosuppressant used often in combination with CNIs and steroids. MMF was introduced in 1995 and has largely replaced azathioprine in transplantation, as clinical trials showed superiority of MMF when compared to azathioprine. [29] Based on a recent SRTR report in 2009, MMF was part of the initial maintenance regimen in 89.9% of kidney transplant recipients.

6.7. Mechanism of action

Mycophenolate mofetil is an inactive prodrug with mycophenolic acid (MPA) being its active component. The mofetil entity significantly increases bioavailability of MPA. There is an enteric coated form of MPA also available for use that may be better tolerated in some patients. MPA is a selective, reversible inhibitor of inosine monophosphate dehydrogenase (IMPDH) which is the rate-limiting enzyme in the denovo synthesis of purines. T- and B-lymphocytes are more dependent on this pathway than other cell types for proliferation since they do not have a salvage pathway for purine synthesis. Moreover, MPA is a more potent inhibitor of the type II isoform of IMPDH, which is predominatly expressed in activated lymphocytes.

6.8. Clinical use

MMF was initially approved for standard dose administration of 1 gram twice daily in adult kidney transplant recipients. Therapeutic drug monitoring for MMF/MPA is not performed routinely since several factors can impact the MPA AUC (detailed in the section below). Recent studies however have shown an association between MPA exposure and clinical outcomes (rejection and toxicity) and therapeutic drug monitoring (TDM) in certain circumstances may be warranted. [30] [31] The APOMYGRE study has shown decreased incidence of acute rejection with individualized MMF dosing based on drug exposure. [32]

When a serious infection develops, MMF or MPA is typically held since the drug's impact on lymphocyte proliferation is reversible and the immunosuppressive effects disappear within a few days. Intravenous formulations are available for MMF and intravenous dosing is the same as oral dosing with 1:1 conversion. Dose adjustment is not necessary in renal insufficiency. These drugs are not dialyzable. Use of MMF in pregnancy is contraindicated since it is associated with congenital malformations in the fetus especially facial abnormalities.[33] Mycophenolate should be discontinued before planned pregnancy in both male and female transplant recipients.

6.9. MMF exposure and metabolism

Mycophenolate moefetil is rapidly absorbed and hydrolysed to yield the active component MPA mainly in the liver, which is detectable in peripheral blood within 1-2 hours. MPA is then converted to 7-0-MPA glucuronide also referred to as MPAG (an inactive metabolite) by UDP-glucuronosyl transferase (UDPGT) in the liver and intestine. MPAG is excreted through the bile and urine. Both MPA and MPAG are protein bound. So factors such as low albumin concentration and high urea levels can decrease protein binding and lead to rapid clearance of the drug. MPAG accumulation in renal failure displaces MPA from protein binding and can lead to an increase in the free fraction of the drug. Once MPAG is excreted in the bile it can be converted back to MPA by bacterial glucuronidases and lead to increased levels of MPA (enterohepatic recirculation). This leads to a second peak in the drug concentration 6 to 12 hours after administration which contributes to more than 30% of the area under the curve. Cyclosporine leads to inhibition of this second peak by blocking the transporters involved in biliary excretion of MPAG. So typically patients on cyclosporine need higher doses of MMF or MPA compared to patients on tacrolimus. Antibiotic therapy is also known to have a similar impact by inhibiting bacterial proliferation in the gut and hence inhibiting enterohepatic recirculation.

There is no significant drug interaction with medications that induce or block the CYP3A pathway. When used in combination with sirolimus both agents can lead to cytopenias. Generally co administration with antacids and cholestyramine should be avoided as they interfere with absorption of MMF.

6.10. Toxicity

The main dose limiting toxicity of MMF or enteric coated MPA is related to gastrointestinal (GI) side effects. More than one third of patients develop diarrhea and in addition some patients have nonspecific GI intolerance in the form of dyspepsia, nausea and vomiting. Indeed, there is evidence demonstrating a correlation between drug exposure and GI toxicity. [31] Most of these side effects are handled with either dose reduction or splitting the dose into 3 to 4 divided doses. Although patients may tolerate enteric coated MPA better, studies curiously do not demonstrate major differences in the GI side effect profile of MMF and enteric coated MPA. [34]

Another major side effect of these preparations is bone marrow suppression mainly manifesting with leucopenia. Typically the dose of MMF is reduced based on the severity of leucopenia. There appears to be a correlation between the incidence of leucopenia and drug exposure. [31] Anemia and thrombocytopenia can occur as well.

6.11. Azathioprine

Azathioprine (Imuran) has been in use in transplantation for more than three decades. With introduction of CNIs and MMF, many centers have moved away from using azathioprine as a first line maintenance agent. SRTR reports from 2009 demonstrate that only 0.6% of the kidney transplant recipients were on Azathioprine. It is commonly used now primarily in patients who are intolerant to MMF. Usual daily dose administered is 2-3 mg/kg once daily.

6.12. Mechanism of action, metabolism and major drug interactions

Azathioprine is an antimetabolite a derivative of 6-mercaptopurine. It gets incorporated into cellular deoxyribonucleic acid (DNA). Once incorporated into DNA it interferes with transcription, purine and ribonucleic acid (RNA) synthesis which are important for T cell activation. Azathioprine is metabolized by xanthine oxidase inhibitor to 6–thiouric acid. Hence allopurinol which is a xanthine oxidase inhibitor should be used with great caution with azathioprine as it can lead to significant toxicity. Typically the dose of azathioprine is reduced when used in combination with allopurinol.

6.13. Adverse drug reactions

The single most severe toxicity of azathioprine is related to suppression of bone marrow. Patients can develop profound leucopenia and thrombocytopenia. It is recommended to monitor white count and platelet count carefully every 2 weeks at initiation. The dose of the drug will need to be decreased if leucopenia occurs and severe leucopenia might necessitate discontinuation of the drug. Cholestasis, hepatic veno occlusive disease, hepatitis and rare cases of pancreatitis have been described with azathioprine use.

6.14. Sirolimus

Sirolimus (Rapamycin) was introduced to transplantation in the late 1990s. It has antitumor, antiproliferative and immunosuppressive actions. Sirolimus plays a key role in immunosuppression especially as an alternative to CNIs to minimize long term CNI induced nephrotoxicity. SRTR database reported that the use of sirolimus as part of initial maintenance regimen peaked in 2001; however it gradually declined to only 3% of kidney transplant recipients receiving it in 2009. In the same report at 1 year post transplantation, 6.5% of recipients were receiving sirolimus. The declining use of sirolimus can be attributed to the side effects encountered with medication usage.

The unique antitumoral properties of sirolimus, however, make it an attractive option for immunosuppression in patients with post transplant malignancies. Recent study reported by Euvrard et al (Tumorapa study) has shown that sirolimus conversion has provided protection against recurrence of skin cancers in patients with squamous cell carcinomas of the skin post transplant. [35]

6.15. Mechanism of action

Similar to CNIs sirolimus binds to cytoplasmic protein FKBP-12 to mediate its action. The sirolimus/FKBP-12 complex then inhibits mTOR (mammalian target of rapamune). This enzyme is a kinase that plays a key role in cell cycle progression (G1-S transition). Blocking mTOR has a profound effect on inhibiting T-cell proliferation and expansion. mTOR is expressed ubiquitously so the antiproliferative effects of sirolimus is not limited to lymphocytes and attributes to several adverse effects of the drug which are detailed below.

The anti-tumor effect of sirolimus is mediated by inhibiting the PI3K-AKT pathway which plays a critical role in cell proliferation, survival, migration and angiogenesis. [36] In addition it inhibits growth of endothelial cells and tumor angiogenesis by interfering with synthesis of vascular endothelial growth factor.

6.16. Clinical use

Sirolimus has a long half life of 60 to 70 hours so consideration is needed when initiating the drug or making dose adjustments. Usually patients receive a loading dose of 3-15mg followed by once daily dosing of 1-5mg per day. The loading and maintenance dose are generally determined by patient weight and immunologic risk. The dose is then adjusted based on drug levels. Therapeutic drug monitoring is routinely used with sirolimus. It is recommended to check 24 hour trough levels several days after initiation or dosage adjustment of sirolimus since it takes longer to achieve a steady state.

The drug is available as oral tablet at 0.5mg, 1mg and 2mgs dose. In addition there is also liquid formulation with strength of 1mg/ml. It is metabolized by CYP3A and hence dose needs to be adjusted in liver disease, but not in renal impairment.

6.17. Metabolism and drug interactions

As both sirolimus and CNIs are metabolized by CYP3A enzyme pathway, concomitant use of both agents can increase exposure to sirolimus 2 to 3 fold. It is generally recommended that sirolimus be administered a few hours after CNI dosing. Similar to CNIs, it interacts with drugs that induce and block the CYP3A pathway. Sirolimus is not renally excreted so dose adjustment is not needed in renal failure. However dose adjustment is recommended in patients with hepatic dysfunction.

6.18. Adverse reactions

Sirolimus is considered to be less nephrotoxic than CNIs, however there are some unique renal side effects related to its use. Sirolimus potentiates CNI nephrotoxicity and can be tubulotoxic leading to hypomagnesemia and hypokalemia. De novo development of proteinuria, or exaggeration of preexisting proteinura is seen with conversion to sirolimus.[37] Use of sirolimus is in fact contraindicated if patient has 24 hour urine protein exceeding 1 gram/day. Sirolimus has been reported to have a direct toxic effect on podocytes. [38] [39] Sirolimus associated cast nephropathy has been reported as well. [40] Thrombotic microangiopathy has also been observed with sirolimus use, likely mediated by its inhibition of VEGF pathway. [41] The discontinuation rate of Sirolimus was as high as 30% in clinical studies due to adverse reactions. [42-44]

Use of sirolimus is not recommended immediately after transplant surgery as sirolimus impairs wound healing (by inhibiting fibroblast proliferation). Sirolimus can increase the risk of lymphocele formation and is also associated with prolonged recovery from delayed graft function. [45]. Due to its effects on tissue repair, sirolimus is generally stopped few weeks prior to any anticipated elective surgery. Metabolic side effects of sirolimus include hyperlipidemia and hyperglycemia. Sirolimus use is also associated with non-infectious atypical pneumonitis. Bactrim is typically prescribed for one year as there are studies observing fatal pneumocystis pneumonia with sirolimus use. Sirolimus also suppresses bone marrow leading to cytopenias. Cell counts should be closely monitored especially when used in combination with MMF. Patients also can develop oral ulcers with this agent.

Adverse Effects	Tac	CsA	mTORi	MMF	Steroids
Nephrotoxicity	↑	↑			
Proteinuria			↑↑		
Hypertension		↑↑			↑↑
Hyperlipidemia		↑	↑↑		↑
New Onset Diabetes	↑↑	↑	↑		↑
Delayed Wound Healing			↑		
Osteopenia	↑	↑			↑↑
Hyperuricemia					
Anemia/Leuko penia			↑	↑	
GI side effects	↑			↑↑	

Tac, Tacrolimus; CsA, Cyclosporine; mTORi, mammalian target of rapamycin inhibitor; MMF, mycophenolate mofetil

↑: mild-moderate adverse effect on the complication

↑↑: moderate-severe adverse effect on the complication

Table 3. Adverse Effects Of Maintenance Immunosuppressive agents

6.19. Everolimus

There are recent studies on use of everolimus in kidney transplant recipients. [46] It is similar to sirolimus in terms of mechanism of action and side effect profile. The only major difference from sirolimus is its shorter half life.

6.20. Corticosteroids

Since the early 1960's, corticosteroids were used in kidney transplantation both as maintenance agents and to treat acute rejections. [47-49]. Corticosteroids down-regulate cytokine gene expression through interference with transcription. Since they are lipophilic they first translocate into cytoplasm and bind to receptors. The steroid –receptor complex then translocates to the nucleus to bind to glucocorticoid responsive elements on DNA to regulate transcription. By dampening cytokine production they blunt the immune response generated by T cells. Long-term steroid use is associated with several adverse effects including hypertension, new onset diabetes after transplantation, osteoporosis, fractures, hyperlipidemia, growth retardation, weight gain, avascular necrosis, cataracts, cosmetic changes, depression, and psychotic behavior. With the advent of potent maintenance and induction agents the transplant community is now moving more and more towards steroid sparing strategies.

6.21. Leflunomide

Leflunomide is used for maintenance immunousppression especially in patients with BK nephropathy. [50, 51] It has both imunosuppressive properties and antiviral activity against BK. It blocks pyramidine synthesis in lymphocytes. The common adverse effects with its use are GI toxicity and neuropathy. There are no major drug interactions with leflunomide.

7. Alternative maintenance regimens

Different immunosuppressive strategies and protocols have evolved over time to address several major concerns with maintenance regimens. Major concerns include the long term side effects of chronic steroid use, as well as long term calcineurin nephrotoxicity which contribute to decreased long-term graft survival. Protocols that have been studied and published include steroid withdrawal and avoidance, as well as studies where calcineurin use is avoided, minimized or replaced with other agents.

7.1. Steroid withdrawal/avoidance (SAW)

Steroid withdrawal typically involves discontinuing steroids several months post transplantation whereas steroid avoidance involves no corticosteroid maintenance at all and only a brief exposure to steroids in the immediate post operative period. Studies demonstrate that early steroid withdrawal is safer than late withdrawal as late withdrawal was associated with increased risk of acute rejections. [52, 53] A recent meta-analysis of 34 randomized controlled studies using SAW regimens published by Knight et al concluded that SAW is associated with increased risk of acute rejection, however this did not impact long term patient or graft survival. [54] There is a more favorable cardiovascular profile with SAW most likely secondary to decreased incidence of hypertension, new onset diabetes and dyslipidemia. As many studies have shown increased risk of acute rejections with SAW it is generally implemented with caution in high immunologic risk recipients (high PRA, repeat transplants, young African American recipients, patients with prior rejections and/or unstable graft function). With use of more potent induction regimens more US centers are currently implementing SAW in immunologically low risk recipients.

7.2. Calcineurin inhibitor avoidance/minimization/withdrawal

Several studies have looked at minimizing exposure to CNIs to over come nephrotoxicity. Complete calcineurin avoidance with de novo use of sirolimus has not been successful and was associated with higher incidence of rejections and graft loss. [43]. Due to this, more centers and studies have favored calcineurin minimization and withdrawal (at 3 to 6 months post transplant) as opposed to complete avoidance. The ELITE-symphony trial was a land mark trial comparing different regimens of calcineurin minimization and withdrawal demonstrating better allograft outcomes at three years of follow up in patients on low dose tacrolimus (in addition to steroids and MMF) than standard dose cyclosporine, reduced dose cyclosporine or low dose sirolimus as primary maintenance agent. [44] A recent meta-analysis evaluating calcineurin minimization strategies concluded that calcineurin minimization decreases rates of graft failure, incidence of delayed graft function, and new onset diabetes post transplant while avoiding an increased risk of acute rejection. [55].

8. Antirejection therapies

Rejection is a common problem with renal allografts, and can be of cellular (lymphocyte) and/ or humoral (circulating antibody) origin. It is well known that if acute rejection is left untreated, eventually graft failure ensues. Rejection can be acute or subclinical. Acute rejection is clinically evident and often presents as a decline in kidney function associated with a rise in creatinine and classic histologic changes seen on renal biopsy. On the other hand, subclinical rejection is subtle; where histologic changes of rejection may be present in grafts that otherwise appear to have stable renal function. Immunosuppressive management for subclinical rejection has not been well delineated. [56-58] Finally, rejection may be mixed and have both cellular and humoral components.

Overall the incidence of acute rejection post-transplant has decreased. However, survival of allografts has not increased to the extent predicted, mostly due to the universal development of chronic allograft dysfunction and late graft loss. Chronic allo-immune injury has been recognized as a major contributor to late graft loss and can present early on in transplantation as demonstrated by several protocol biopsy studies. [59, 60] Compared to cell-mediated rejections, humoral rejection and chronic rejection can be challenging to treat. In addition, the optimal treatments for humoral rejection, subclinical rejection and chronic rejection have yet to be defined by the transplant community..

8.1. Treatment of cellular rejection

Acute cellular rejection is a T-cell–mediated process, is usually easy to treat, and responds well to therapy. T-cell directed induction therapies, and calcineurin maintenance has substantially decreased the overall incidence of cell-mediated acute rejections. Low grade cellular rejection with out vascular involvement is treated with high dose, intravenous steroids. The dose and duration of treatment with corticosteroids has not been well defined by studies, and is often left to physician discretion. Thymoglobulin in combination with steroids is used to treat severe and high grade acute cellular rejections with a vascular component. Although Thymoglobulin is most widely used for high grade cellular rejections, there are small case series and small studies that favor the use of alemtuzumab for treatment of cellular rejections. [61]

8.2. Treatment of humoral rejection

Humoral rejection mediated by alloreactive B-cells, alloantibodies and complement are more challenging to treat. Humoral rejection is often refractory to treatment and continues to be a significant problem in transplantation due to difficulties in establishing a consensus for safe optimal treatments directed against allosensitization and alloantibody production. Humoral responses also greatly contribute to late acute graft losses and the development of chronic rejection. [62] Humoral rejection has been linked to the presence of donor specific antibody and activation of complement resulting in C4d deposits in renal tissue. Therapeutic strategies have been aimed both at removing alloantibodies as well as decreasing alloantibody production by impairing and/or depleting B-cells. [63, 64]

The best known treatment algorithms to treat antibody mediated rejection include combinations of plasma exchange to remove donor-specific antibody, and/or intravenous immunoglobulins and the anti-CD20 monoclonal antibody (rituximab) to suppress donor-specific antibody production. [65, 66] There are no randomized controlled trials powered to show efficacy or safety of potential different combinations of these different therapeutic strategies. Some side effects of plasmapheresis include hypotension, citrate induced hypocalcemia, complications with access placement, and infections due to removal of immunoglobulins. Adverse reactions of IVIG include anaphylactoid reactions, fevers, chills, flushing, myalgias, malaise, headache, nausea, vomiting, dilutional hyponatremia, pseudohyponatremia, hemolysis and neutropenia. See previous section on Rituximab for side effects.

Bortezomib continues to be a promising agent for acute humoral rejection because of its ability to target multiple pathways involved in B-cell activation and antibody production and its direct activity against CD138+ long lived plasma cells that exist in survival niches such as the bone marrow and spleen. [67] These cells, primarily responsible for producing high affinity alloantibody, are not targeted by Rituximab, the current mainstay treatment for humoral rejection. [68, 69] Initial reports on Bortezomib were in patients with AMR that were refractory to traditional anti-humoral therapies, but recent reports show that Bortezomib can be used as primary therapy for AMR. [70] In terms of its ability to decrease the levels of donor specific antibodies in sensitized patients and patients with AMR, studies have provided mixed results. [71, 72] Part of this may be secondary to differing conditioning regimens that accompany the use of Bortezomib. Another important finding reported by two studies is the differential responses of early versus late AMR after treatment with Bortezomib, with early AMR responding much better than late. [25]

8.3. Treatment of mixed rejection

Rejection may be mixed and have both cellular and humoral components. To date, there are no randomized control studies evaluating different therapies for the treatment of mixed rejection. Case series and small studies suggest that choosing a biologic agent that has activity against both T-cell and B-cell activity would be more favorable. Agents that have broad based activity such as Campath or Bortezomib may be better choices, than T-cell directed agents such as rATG. Plasmapharesis and IVIG may also be added therapies, especially if there is the presence of circulating donor specific antibody. Unfortunately, trials evaluating different combinations of these therapies or head to head comparison of these biologic agents do not exist.

9. Novel immunosuppressive agents

Given substantially decreased rates of acute rejection secondary to potent induction agents and CNI based maintenance regimens, the focus has shifted away from acute rejection to preserving grafts for the long-term. However, many studies are still focused on short term outcomes and there are very few studies looking at which drugs or combinations thereof offer better long term graft function.

Long term graft preservation may be particularly challenging given the nephrotoxic effects of CNIs on allografts. To address this issue, a number of novel agents are undergoing trials currently as a replacement to CNIs. [73] Several biologic agents and fusion proteins have emerged and unfortunately many of these agents have been discarded after preliminary trials due to their toxicity. In addition there are several trials focusing on tolerogenic protocols to avoid use of long term immunosuppression. Table 4 below summarizes the new agents that are currently undergoing clinical trials. Belatacept discussed below, is a newer biologic agent that has been studied the most extensively.

9.1. Belatacept

Belatacept is a recombinant fusion protein with an extracellular domain that consists of human cytotoxic T lymphocyte antigen-4 (CTLA-4) and the Fc fragment of human IgG. The fusion protein Belatacept (CTLA-4Ig) blocks the interaction of CD80/86 present on antigen presenting cells (APC), with the CD28 receptor expressed on T cells. CD80/86 are costimulatory molecules that are necessary for providing costimulation and full activation of T-cells, a requirement for T-cell cytokine production and expansion. The most exciting feature of CTLA4Ig is its known ability to generate immune tolerance particularly in animal models of transplantation and autoimmunity. [74, 75] Whether tolerance can be generated in vivo in humans, however remains to be seen.

Agent	Mechanism of action	Clinical Indication	Studies
TOL101	Target ? T-cell receptor Non-depletional Inactivates Tcell	Induction	Phase 2
Sotrastaurin	Proteinkinase C inhibitor Blocks T-cell activation	Maintenance	Studies halted secondary to increased rejection rates
Tofacitinib	Inhibitor of the JAK/STAT pathway. Blocks T-cell activation	Maintenance	Phase 2
ASKP1240	Humanized antibody against CD40 on antigen presenting cells	Maintenance	Phase 1

*References [77-79]

Table 4. Novel Immunosuppressive Agents

Belatacept is a relatively new agent used in human transplantation with the first report of its use in human renal transplantation in 2005. The focus of clinical investigative trials utilizing belatacept was to provide a new effective maintenance regimen that would allow for the avoidance of the renal and metabolic side effects of chronic CNI use. Studies such as the BENEFIT and BENEFIT-EXT trials demonstrate its efficacy as a maintenance agent in place of calcineurin inhibitors. [76] The three year follow up data of BENEFIT where belatacept was compared to cyclosporine concluded that patient and graft survival were comparable with better GFR in the belatacept arm. There was however increased incidence of acute rejection and early post transplant lymphoproliferative disease in the belatacept group (especially in EBV sero negative patients). For this reason, belatacept use is approved only for patients who are EBV seropositive. The cost and long term need for intravenous administration of the drug appear to be major obstacles for wide spread use of belatacept. Nevertheless, it still provides a valuable alternative to long term CNI use.

10. Conclusion

Establishing optimal immunosuppressive regimens involves maintaining a delicate balance between over-immunosuppression which increases infection risk and under-immunosuppression which increases risk of allograft rejection. Use of potent induction agents and maintenance therapies that include CNI has led to dramatic decrease in the incidence of acute rejection episodes in the immediate post transplantation period. However, late allograft loss and long-term graft survival are problems that persist despite better immunosuppression. Chronic CNI toxicity, humoral rejection and the development of chronic alloreactivity to donor allograft tissue are major contributing factors to late graft loss.

One challenge with current maintenance regimens is the toxicity related to long term CNI use. Steroid avoidance/withdrawal protocols continue to be evaluated and are being implemented successfully at some centers. Rapamune has been studied in several trials as a CNI sparing agent, but has not gained wide acceptance due to its side effect profile. The predominant trend in recent clinical trials is to find a long term alternative agent to replace CNI. Belatacept was recently approved by the FDA for use as maintenance agent and appears to be a promising alternative to long term CNI use. However, the majority of centers lack experience with belatacept and long term outcome data is lacking.

Other challenges include the rising percentage of sensitized patients on the transplant wait list. Strategies to offer transplantation to these highly sensitized recipients include transplantation against a positive cross match donor, paired kidney exchange and aggressive desensitization to lower alloantibody titers. Immunosuppressive protocols aimed at successfully transplanting sensitized recipients continue to be investigated as these patients present a special immunologic challenge. Sensitized patients are at increased risk of developing antibody mediated rejection and earlier graft loss post-transplant. Several new agents like bortezomib and eculizumab are currently being tested in these patients.

Finally, the optimal immunosuppressive strategy would ideally be one which promotes the development of tolerance to alloantigens such that immunosuppression can be withdrawn successfully. The development of tolerance is certainly possible as the literature supports incidental cases of operational tolerance, where recipients are on minimal or no immunosuppression without evidence of allograft rejection. Currently, the majority of patients will require life long immunosuppressive therapy. Basic mechanisms promoting tolerance are being investigated with the hope that new medications or tolerogenic protocols may be implemented in the near future.

Author details

M. Ghanta, J. Dreier, R. Jacob and I. Lee*

*Address all correspondence to: iris.lee@tuhs.temple.edu

Section of Nephrology, Temple University School of Medicine, Philadelphia, PA, USA

References

[1] Lamb, K. E, & Lodhi, S. Meier-Kriesche HU: Long-term renal allograft survival in the United States: a critical reappraisal. Am J Transplant, , 11, 450-462.

[2] Einecke, G, Sis, B, Reeve, J, Mengel, M, Campbell, P. M, Hidalgo, L. G, & Kaplan, B. Halloran PF: Antibody-mediated microcirculation injury is the major cause of late kidney transplant failure. Am J Transplant (2009).

[3] Cai, J. Terasaki PI: Induction immunosuppression improves long-term graft and patient outcome in organ transplantation: an analysis of United Network for Organ Sharing registry data. Transplantation, , 90, 1511-1515.

[4] Beiras-fernandez, A, & Thein, E. Hammer C: Induction of immunosuppression with polyclonal antithymocyte globulins: an overview. Exp Clin Transplant (2003).

[5] Zand, M. S, Vo, T, Huggins, J, Felgar, R, Liesveld, J, Pellegrin, T, Bozorgzadeh, A, & Sanz, I. Briggs BJ: Polyclonal rabbit antithymocyte globulin triggers B-cell and plasma cell apoptosis by multiple pathways. Transplantation (2005).

[6] Lopez, M, Clarkson, M. R, Albin, M, Sayegh, M. H, & Najafian, N. A novel mechanism of action for anti-thymocyte globulin: induction of CD4+CD25+Foxp3+ regulatory T cells. J Am Soc Nephrol (2006).

[7] Stock, P. G, Barin, B, Murphy, B, Hanto, D, Diego, J. M, Light, J, Davis, C, Blumberg, E, Simon, D, Subramanian, A, et al. Outcomes of kidney transplantation in HIV-infected recipients. N Engl J Med, (2004). , 363, 2004-2014.

[8] Trullas, J. C, Cofan, F, Tuset, M, Ricart, M. J, Brunet, M, Cervera, C, Manzardo, C, Lopez-dieguez, M, Oppenheimer, F, Moreno, A, et al. Renal transplantation in HIV-infected patients: (2010). update. Kidney Int, , 79, 825-842.

[9] Kamar, N, Borde, J. S, Sandres-saune, K, Suc, B, Barange, K, Cointault, O, Lavayssiere, L, Durand, D, & Izopet, J. Rostaing L: Induction therapy with either anti-CD25 monoclonal antibodies or rabbit antithymocyte globulins in liver transplantation for hepatitis C. Clin Transplant (2005).

[10] Roth, D, Gaynor, J. J, Reddy, K. R, Ciancio, G, Sageshima, J, Kupin, W, Guerra, G, Chen, L, & Burke, G. W. rd: Effect of kidney transplantation on outcomes among patients with hepatitis C. J Am Soc Nephrol, , 22, 1152-1160.

[11] Noel, C, Abramowicz, D, Durand, D, Mourad, G, Lang, P, Kessler, M, Charpentier, B, Touchard, G, Berthoux, F, Merville, P, et al. Daclizumab versus antithymocyte globulin in high-immunological-risk renal transplant recipients. J Am Soc Nephrol (2009).

[12] Locke, J. E, Montgomery, R. A, Warren, D. S, & Subramanian, A. Segev DL: Renal transplant in HIV-positive patients: long-term outcomes and risk factors for graft loss. Arch Surg (2009).

[13] Carter, J. T, Melcher, M. L, Carlson, L. L, & Roland, M. E. Stock PG: Thymoglobulin-associated Cd4+ T-cell depletion and infection risk in HIV-infected renal transplant recipients. Am J Transplant (2006).

[14] (Hanaway MJ, Woodle ES, Mulgaonkar S, Peddi VR, Kaufman DB, First MR, Croy R, Holman J: Alemtuzumab induction in renal transplantation. N Engl J Med, 364:1909-1919). 364, 1909-1919.

[15] Vo, A. A, Lukovsky, M, Toyoda, M, Wang, J, Reinsmoen, N. L, Lai, C. H, Peng, A, & Villicana, R. Jordan SC: Rituximab and intravenous immune globulin for desensitization during renal transplantation. N Engl J Med (2008).

[16] Takagi, T, Ishida, H, Shirakawa, H, & Shimizu, T. Tanabe K: Evaluation of low-dose rituximab induction therapy in living related kidney transplantation. Transplantation, , 89, 1466-1470.

[17] Clatworthy, M. R, Watson, C. J, Plotnek, G, Bardsley, V, Chaudhry, A. N, & Bradley, J. A. Smith KG: B-cell-depleting induction therapy and acute cellular rejection. N Engl J Med (2009).

[18] (Stegall MD, Diwan T, Raghavaiah S, Cornell LD, Burns J, Dean PG, Cosio FG, Gandhi MJ, Kremers W, Gloor JM: Terminal complement inhibition decreases antibody-mediated rejection in sensitized renal transplant recipients. Am J Transplant, 11:2405-2413). 11, 2405-2413.

[19] Perry, D. K, Burns, J. M, Pollinger, H. S, Amiot, B. P, Gloor, J. M, & Gores, G. J. Stegall MD: Proteasome inhibition causes apoptosis of normal human plasma cells preventing alloantibody production. Am J Transplant (2009).

[20] Wu J: On the role of proteasomes in cell biology and proteasome inhibition as a novel frontier in the development of immunosuppressants. (2002). *Am J Transplant.*

[21] Wang, X, Luo, H, Chen, H, & Duguid, W. Wu J: Role of proteasomes in T cell activation and proliferation. J Immunol (1998).

[22] Everly, M. J, Everly, J. J, Susskind, B, Brailey, P, Arend, L. J, Alloway, R. R, Roychaudhury, P, Govil, A, Mogilishetty, G, Rike, A. H, et al. Bortezomib provides effective therapy for antibody- and cell-mediated acute rejection. Transplantation (2008).

[23] Idica, A, Kaneku, H, Everly, M. J, Trivedi, H. L, Feroz, A, Vanikar, A. V, Shankar, V, Trivedi, V. B, Modi, P. R, Khemchandani, S. I, et al. Elimination of post-transplant donor-specific HLA antibodies with bortezomib. Clin Transpl (2008). , 2008, 229-239.

[24] Lee, I, Constantinescu, S, Gillespie, A, Swami, A, Birkenbach, M, Leech, S, Silva, P, Karachristos, A, & Daller, J. A. Sifontis NM: Bortezomib as therapy for mixed humoral and cellular rejection: should it be first line? Clin Transpl (2009). , 2009, 425-429.

[25] Lee, I, Constantinescu, S, Gillespie, A, Rao, S, Silva, P, Birkenbach, M, Leech, S, Karachristos, A, & Daller, J. A. Sifontis NM: Targeting alloantibody production with bortezomib: does it make more sense? Clin Transpl:, 397-403.

[26] Madsen, K, Friis, U. G, Gooch, J. L, Hansen, P. B, Holmgaard, L, & Skott, O. Jensen BL: Inhibition of calcineurin phosphatase promotes exocytosis of renin from juxtaglomerular cells. Kidney Int, , 77, 110-117.

[27] Khanna, A. K, Cairns, V. R, & Becker, C. G. Hosenpud JD: Transforming growth factor (TGF)-beta mimics and anti-TGF-beta antibody abrogates the in vivo effects of cyclosporine: demonstration of a direct role of TGF-beta in immunosuppression and nephrotoxicity of cyclosporine. Transplantation (1999).

[28] Wu, Q, Marescaux, C, Wolff, V, Jeung, M. Y, Kessler, R, & Lauer, V. Chen Y: Tacrolimus-associated posterior reversible encephalopathy syndrome after solid organ transplantation. Eur Neurol, , 64, 169-177.

[29] Meier-kriesche, H. U, Steffen, B. J, Hochberg, A. M, Gordon, R. D, Liebman, M. N, & Morris, J. A. Kaplan B: Mycophenolate mofetil versus azathioprine therapy is associated with a significant protection against long-term renal allograft function deterioration. Transplantation (2003).

[30] Hale, M. D, Nicholls, A. J, Bullingham, R. E, Hene, R, Hoitsma, A, Squifflet, J. P, Weimar, W, & Vanrenterghem, Y. Van de Woude FJ, Verpooten GA: The pharmacokinetic-pharmacodynamic relationship for mycophenolate mofetil in renal transplantation. Clin Pharmacol Ther (1998).

[31] Van Gelder, T, Hilbrands, L. B, Vanrenterghem, Y, Weimar, W, De Fijter, J. W, Squifflet, J. P, Hene, R. J, Verpooten, G. A, Navarro, M. T, Hale, M. D, & Nicholls, A. J. A randomized double-blind, multicenter plasma concentration controlled study of the safety and efficacy of oral mycophenolate mofetil for the prevention of acute rejection after kidney transplantation. Transplantation (1999).

[32] Le Meur YBuchler M, Thierry A, Caillard S, Villemain F, Lavaud S, Etienne I, Westeel PF, Hurault de Ligny B, Rostaing L, et al: Individualized mycophenolate mofetil dosing based on drug exposure significantly improves patient outcomes after renal transplantation. Am J Transplant (2007).

[33] Coscia, L. A, Constantinescu, S, Moritz, M. J, Frank, A. M, Ramirez, C. B, Maley, W. R, Doria, C, & Mcgrory, C. H. Armenti VT: Report from the National Transplantation Pregnancy Registry (NTPR): outcomes of pregnancy after transplantation. Clin Transpl:, 65-85.

[34] Cooper, M, Deering, K. L, Slakey, D. P, Harshaw, Q, Arcona, S, Mccann, E. L, & Rasetto, F. A. Florman SS: Comparing outcomes associated with dose manipulations of enteric-coated mycophenolate sodium versus mycophenolate mofetil in renal transplant recipients. Transplantation (2009).

[35] Euvrard, S, Morelon, E, Rostaing, L, Goffin, E, Brocard, A, Tromme, I, & Broeders, N. del Marmol V, Chatelet V, Dompmartin A, et al: Sirolimus and secondary skin-cancer prevention in kidney transplantation. N Engl J Med, , 367, 329-339.

[36] Dormond, O, & Madsen, J. C. Briscoe DM: The effects of mTOR-Akt interactions on anti-apoptotic signaling in vascular endothelial cells. J Biol Chem (2007).

[37] Dogan, E, & Ghanta, M. Tanriover B: Collapsing glomerulopathy in a renal transplant recipient: potential molecular mechanisms. Ann Transplant, , 16, 113-116.

[38] (Biancone L, Bussolati B, Mazzucco G, Barreca A, Gallo E, Rossetti M, Messina M, Nuschak B, Fop F, Medica D, et al: Loss of nephrin expression in glomeruli of kidney-transplanted patients under m-TOR inhibitor therapy. Am J Transplant, 10:2270-2278). 10, 2270-2278.

[39] Stallone, G, Infante, B, Pontrelli, P, Gigante, M, Montemurno, E, Loverre, A, Rossini, M, Schena, F. P, & Grandaliano, G. Gesualdo L: Sirolimus and proteinuria in renal transplant patients: evidence for a dose-dependent effect on slit diaphragm-associated proteins. Transplantation, , 91, 997-1004.

[40] Coombes, J. D, Mreich, E, & Liddle, C. Rangan GK: Rapamycin worsens renal function and intratubular cast formation in protein overload nephropathy. Kidney Int (2005).

[41] Reynolds, J. C, Agodoa, L. Y, & Yuan, C. M. Abbott KC: Thrombotic microangiopathy after renal transplantation in the United States. Am J Kidney Dis (2003).

[42] Lebranchu, Y, Thierry, A, Toupance, O, Westeel, P. F, Etienne, I, Thervet, E, Moulin, B, & Frouget, T. Le Meur Y, Glotz D, et al: Efficacy on renal function of early conversion from cyclosporine to sirolimus 3 months after renal transplantation: concept study. Am J Transplant (2009).

[43] Glotz, D, Charpentier, B, Abramovicz, D, Lang, P, Rostaing, L, Rifle, G, Vanrenterghem, Y, Berthoux, F, Bourbigot, B, Delahousse, M, et al. Thymoglobulin induction and sirolimus versus tacrolimus in kidney transplant recipients receiving mycophenolate mofetil and steroids. Transplantation, , 89, 1511-1517.

[44] Ekberg, H, Tedesco-silva, H, Demirbas, A, Vitko, S, Nashan, B, Gurkan, A, Margreiter, R, Hugo, C, Grinyo, J. M, Frei, U, et al. Reduced exposure to calcineurin inhibitors in renal transplantation. N Engl J Med (2007).

[45] Mctaggart, R. A, Tomlanovich, S, Bostrom, A, & Roberts, J. P. Feng S: Comparison of outcomes after delayed graft function: sirolimus-based versus other calcineurin-inhibitor sparing induction immunosuppression regimens. Transplantation (2004).

[46] Mjornstedt, L, & Sorensen, S. S. von Zur Muhlen B, Jespersen B, Hansen JM, Bistrup C, Andersson H, Gustafsson B, Undset LH, Fagertun H, et al: Improved Renal Function After Early Conversion From a Calcineurin Inhibitor to Everolimus: a Randomized Trial in Kidney Transplantation. Am J Transplant.

[47] Goodwin, W. E, & Mims, M. M. Kaufman JJ: Human renal transplantation III. Technical problems encountered in six cases of kidney homotransplantation. Trans Am Assoc Genitourin Surg (1962).

[48] Starzl, T. E, & Marchioro, T. L. Waddell WR: The Reversal of Rejection in Human Renal Homografts with Subsequent Development of Homograft Tolerance. Surg Gynecol Obstet (1963).

[49] Mcgeown, M. G, Douglas, J. F, Brown, W. A, Donaldson, R. A, Kennedy, J. A, Loughridge, W. G, & Mehta, S. Hill CM: Low dose steroid from the day following renal transplantation. Proc Eur Dial Transplant Assoc (1979).

[50] Josephson, M. A, Gillen, D, Javaid, B, Kadambi, P, Meehan, S, Foster, P, Harland, R, Thistlethwaite, R. J, Garfinkel, M, Atwood, W, et al. Treatment of renal allograft polyoma BK virus infection with leflunomide. Transplantation (2006).

[51] Williams, J. W, Javaid, B, Kadambi, P. V, Gillen, D, Harland, R, Thistlewaite, J. R, Garfinkel, M, Foster, P, Atwood, W, Millis, J. M, et al. Leflunomide for polyomavirus type BK nephropathy. N Engl J Med (2005).

[52] Kasiske, B. L, Chakkera, H. A, Louis, T. A, & Ma, J. Z. A meta-analysis of immunosuppression withdrawal trials in renal transplantation. J Am Soc Nephrol (2000).

[53] Pascual, J, Quereda, C, & Zamora, J. Hernandez D: Steroid withdrawal in renal transplant patients on triple therapy with a calcineurin inhibitor and mycophenolate mofetil: a meta-analysis of randomized, controlled trials. Transplantation (2004).

[54] Knight, S. R. Morris PJ: Steroid avoidance or withdrawal in renal transplantation. Transplantation, 91:e25; author reply e, 26-27.

[55] (Sharif A, Shabir S, Chand S, Cockwell P, Ball S, Borrows R: Meta-analysis of calcineurin-inhibitor-sparing regimens in kidney transplantation. J Am Soc Nephrol, 22:2107-2118). 22, 2107-2118.

[56] Rush, D, Nickerson, P, Gough, J, Mckenna, R, Grimm, P, Cheang, M, Trpkov, K, & Solez, K. Jeffery J: Beneficial effects of treatment of early subclinical rejection: a randomized study. J Am Soc Nephrol (1998).

[57] Rush, D. N, Karpinski, M. E, Nickerson, P, Dancea, S, & Birk, P. Jeffery JR: Does subclinical rejection contribute to chronic rejection in renal transplant patients? Clin Transplant (1999).

[58] Kurtkoti, J, Sakhuja, V, Sud, K, Minz, M, Nada, R, Kohli, H. S, Gupta, K. L, & Joshi, K. Jha V: The utility of and 3-month protocol biopsies on renal allograft function: a randomized controlled study. Am J Transplant (2008). , 1.

[59] Joosten, S. A, Sijpkens, Y. W, & Van Kooten, C. Paul LC: Chronic renal allograft rejection: pathophysiologic considerations. Kidney Int (2005).

[60] Mengel, M, Chapman, J. R, Cosio, F. G, Cavaille-coll, M. W, Haller, H, Halloran, P. F, Kirk, A. D, Mihatsch, M. J, Nankivell, B. J, Racusen, L. C, et al. Protocol biopsies in renal transplantation: insights into patient management and pathogenesis. Am J Transplant (2007).

[61] Webster, A. C, Pankhurst, T, Rinaldi, F, & Chapman, J. R. Craig JC: Monoclonal and polyclonal antibody therapy for treating acute rejection in kidney transplant recipients: a systematic review of randomized trial data. Transplantation (2006).

[62] Bartel, G, Regele, H, Wahrmann, M, Huttary, N, Exner, M, & Horl, W. H. Bohmig GA: Posttransplant HLA alloreactivity in stable kidney transplant recipients-incidences and impact on long-term allograft outcomes. Am J Transplant (2008).

[63] Terasaki, P. I. Ozawa M: Predicting kidney graft failure by HLA antibodies: a prospective trial. Am J Transplant (2004).

[64] Everly, M. J, Everly, J. J, Arend, L. J, Brailey, P, Susskind, B, Govil, A, Rike, A, Roy-chaudhury, P, Mogilishetty, G, Alloway, R. R, et al. Reducing de novo donor-specific antibody levels during acute rejection diminishes renal allograft loss. Am J Transplant (2009).

[65] Lehrich, R. W, Rocha, P. N, Reinsmoen, N, Greenberg, A, Butterly, D. W, & Howell, D. N. Smith SR: Intravenous immunoglobulin and plasmapheresis in acute humoral rejection: experience in renal allograft transplantation. Hum Immunol (2005).

[66] Levine, M. H. Abt PL: Treatment options and strategies for antibody mediated rejection after renal transplantation. Semin Immunol, , 24, 136-142.

[67] Ellyard, J. I, Avery, D. T, Phan, T. G, Hare, N. J, & Hodgkin, P. D. Tangye SG: Antigen-selected, immunoglobulin-secreting cells persist in human spleen and bone marrow. Blood (2004).

[68] Ramos, E. J, Pollinger, H. S, Stegall, M. D, Gloor, J. M, & Dogan, A. Grande JP: The effect of desensitization protocols on human splenic B-cell populations in vivo. Am J Transplant (2007).

[69] Faguer, S, Kamar, N, Guilbeaud-frugier, C, Fort, M, Modesto, A, Mari, A, Ribes, D, Cointault, O, Lavayssiere, L, Guitard, J, et al. Rituximab therapy for acute humoral rejection after kidney transplantation. Transplantation (2007).

[70] Everly, M. J. A summary of bortezomib use in transplantation across 29 centers. Clin Transpl (2009). , 2009, 323-337.

[71] Trivedi, H. L, Terasaki, P. I, Feroz, A, Everly, M. J, Vanikar, A. V, Shankar, V, Trivedi, V. B, Kaneku, H, Idica, A. K, Modi, P. R, et al. Abrogation of anti-HLA antibodies via proteasome inhibition. Transplantation (2009).

[72] Sberro-soussan, R, Zuber, J, Suberbielle-boissel, C, Candon, S, Martinez, F, Snanoudj, R, Rabant, M, Pallet, N, Nochy, D, Anglicheau, D, et al. Bortezomib as the sole post-

renal transplantation desensitization agent does not decrease donor-specific anti-HLA antibodies. Am J Transplant, , 10, 681-686.

[73] Webber, A, & Hirose, R. Vincenti F: Novel strategies in immunosuppression: issues in perspective. Transplantation, , 91, 1057-1064.

[74] Martin, S. T, & Tichy, E. M. Gabardi S: Belatacept: a novel biologic for maintenance immunosuppression after renal transplantation. Pharmacotherapy, , 31, 394-407.

[75] Sayegh MH: FinallyCTLA4Ig graduates to the clinic. J Clin Invest (1999).

[76] Vincenti, F, Charpentier, B, Vanrenterghem, Y, Rostaing, L, Bresnahan, B, Darji, P, Massari, P, Mondragon-ramirez, G. A, & Agarwal, M. Di Russo G, et al: A phase III study of belatacept-based immunosuppression regimens versus cyclosporine in renal transplant recipients (BENEFIT study). Am J Transplant, , 10, 535-546.

[77] Vincenti, F. Tedesco Silva H, Busque S, O'Connell P, Friedewald J, Cibrik D, Budde K, Yoshida A, Cohney S, Weimar W, et al: Randomized Phase 2b Trial of Tofacitinib (CP-690,550) in De Novo Kidney Transplant Patients: Efficacy, Renal Function and Safety at 1 Year. Am J Transplant.

[78] Oura, T, Yamashita, K, Suzuki, T, Fukumori, D, Watanabe, M, Hirokata, G, Wakayama, K, Taniguchi, M, Shimamura, T, Miura, T, et al. Long-Term Hepatic Allograft Acceptance Based on CD40 Blockade by ASKP1240 in Nonhuman Primates. Am J Transplant, , 12, 1740-1754.

Chapter 5

Hepatitis C Infection in Kidney Transplantion

A.A. Amir, R.A. Amir and S.S. Sheikh

Additional information is available at the end of the chapter

1. Introduction

Hepatitis C is one of the commonest chronic viral infections world-wide and has major health-care implications. According to World Health Organization (WHO), the estimated prevalence of chronic HCV infection world-wide ranges from 0.1% to more than 12%, equating to approximately 170 million chronic carriers and incidence of 3-4 million new cases per year (Carbone et al., 2011). Chronic kidney disease (CKD) in general is present in approximately 10% of the population with many of these patients requiring renal replacement therapy in the form of dialysis and or kidney transplant. A major cause of morbidity and mortality in dialysis patients and kidney transplant recipients is liver disease secondary to hepatitis C virus (HCV) infection. The prevalence of HCV infection is high among renal transplant donors, recipients, and in end stage renal disease (ESRD) patients on dialysis. When HCV infection is present in this group of patients, it has major implications (Scott et al., 2010; Goodkin et al., 2003; Carbone et al., 2011). The major factors associated with this increased relative risk of HCV infection in dialysis patients as opposed to general population are overall exposure of blood products, age, and duration of dialysis (Periera & Levey, 1997; Finelli et al., 2005; Fissell et al., 2004). On the other hand, some recent reports indicate possible decline in prevalence of HCV infection in dialysis patients (Carbone et al., 2011; Scott et al., 2010; Finelli et al., 2005; Fissell et al., 2004; Jadoul et al., 2004; Fribrizi et al., 2002). This decline could be related to the use of erythropoiesis-stimulating agents that consequently lead to decrease in blood transfusions, and progressive enhancement of dialysis conditions to control infections. In developed countries, the prevalence of HCV infection is higher in renal transplant recipients than in dialysis patients, major contributing factors being longer survival of the former with more exposure to blood products, and most probably dialysis.

2. Natural history of HCV infection, morbidity and mortality in transplant

HCV RNA can be detected in the blood after 1-3 weeks of first exposure. In majority of the HCV acute infection cases the patients are asymptomatic, however the disease can have a fulminant course. The natural history of Hepatitis C infection is quite variable with disease spectrum varying from mild to severe hepatitis, hepatic cirrhosis, and hepatocellular carcinoma. In 60-85% of these cases, HCV RNA can be detected for 6 months or longer. 10-15% of these chronic patients progress to develop liver cirrhosis (National Institute of Health [NIH], 2002). The virus is very slow to progress with almost no signs or symptoms in the first few years or decade. The most reliable tool to examine the progression of HCV liver damage is histologic evaluation of liver biopsy. The activity of liver disease can fluctuate, however, once there is fibrosis the damage is considered to be irreversible and progressive. Poynard, in 2001, reported that the average time of HCV infection to progress to liver cirrhosis is about 30 years, ranging from 13 years (for men who drank and were infected after the age of 40 years) to 42 years (for women who did not drink and were infected before the age of 40) (Poynard et al., 2001).

HCV infection has been associated independently with increased mortality in Hemodialysis patients as shown by several studies including Dialysis Outcomes and Practice Patterns (DOPPS) conducted over three continents (Goodkin et al., 2003; Fibrizi, 2004, 2007).

Transplant recipients from HCV positive donors have a higher rate of fulminant or severe hepatitis and liver disease in general. The literature shows some controversy in results presented by various studies regarding survival. The overall survival and specifically of the allograft survival for HCV infected kidney transplant recipients are much worse than non-infected renal transplant recipients (Figures 1 & 2) (Pedroso et al., 2006). Several studies have shown that although recipients of organs from HCV infected donors have higher rates of liver disease, there is no solid evidence of decreased overall survival rate (Periera, 1991, 1995; Mendez et al., 1995). On the other hand, there are some other studies that show contrary results with recipients of organs from HCV infected donors to have significantly higher morbidity mainly due to liver disease and reduced overall survival with limited life expectancy (Pirsch et al., 1995). The presence of liver damage depending on the severity as determined by biopsy is a strong predictor of liver failure and death post-transplantation. Despite the ongoing controversy, majority of the data shows increased morbidity due to higher rate of liver disease. However, there is no consensus on lack of adverse effect on survival by initial studies that mostly represented comparatively small number of cases and short period of followup. Fabrizi and colleagues pooled these single studies in a meta-analysis and showed that anti HCV positive status is an independent and significant risk factor for death and graft failure after kidney transplantation with estimated relative risk of 1.79 and 1.56 respectively. In a recent study, Scott and colleagues also showed prevalence of HCV infection in renal transplant recipients to be 1.8% and reported the patient survival to be 77% and 90% at 5 years and 50% and 79% at 10 years for HCV antibody positive and HCV antibody negative groups. The most common causes of death in HCV positive kidney transplant recipients were cardiovascular disease, malignancy, and liver failure (Scott et al., 2010). In addition to increased mortality, Zylberberg et al found a significantly increased yearly progression rate of liver inflammation and fibrosis in HCV infected renal transplant recipients than immunocompetent group (Zylberberg et al., 2002). Alric and colleagues, on the contrary, showed the annual progression of liver fibrosis to be significantly lower in renal transplant recipients than patients with HCV and normal renal function (Alric et al., 2002). Reasons for the above mentioned difference is not clear. There is strong evidence that transplantation with kidney from HCV infected donor is significantly associated with improved survival as opposed to remaining on dialysis on transplant wait list (Abbott et al., 2004; Periera et al., 1998; Knoll et al., 1997; Maluf et al., 2007). Findings suggest that detrimental effect of transplantation in association with HCV infection does not outweigh its long term benefits on survival in end stage renal disease (ESRD) patients on dialysis and therefore anti-HCV positivity should not be considered as an absolute contraindication for renal transplantation (Natov & Periera, 2012; Knoll et al, 1997).

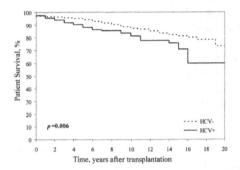

Figure 1. Kaplan-Meier estimate of the cumulative probability of patient survival. Reprinted from Transplantation Proceedings, 38, 1890-1894 (2006), Pedroso S et al., Impact of Hepatitis C Virus on Renal Transplantation: Association with Poor Survival. With permission from Elsevier through Copyright Clearance Center

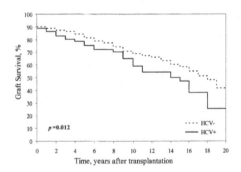

Figure 2. Kaplan-Meier estimate of the cumulative probability of graft survival.Reprinted from Transplantation Proceedings, 38, 1890-1894 (2006), Pedroso S et al., Impact of Hepatitis C Virus on Renal Transplantation: Association with Poor Survival. With permission from Elsevier through Copyright Clearance Center

The increased morbidity and mortality in HCV infection is not only related to liver disease but also extrahepatic complications (Kidney disease: improving global outcome [KDIGO], 2008). HCV infection can predispose to the development of pre and posttransplant diabetes. A 2005 meta-analysis of 2502 patients noted a fourfold increase in the development of New Onset Diabetes mellitus after Transplantation (NODAT) among HCV infected patients when compared to the non-infected group (Gursoy et al., 2000; Abbott et al., 2004). It is suggested that HCV infection might be associated with increased insulin resistance contributing to development of NODAT.

HCV has been associated with renal disease in both native and transplanted kidneys. It is in fact reported to be more associated with glomerular disease in renal transplants than native kidneys. This association is suggested to be secondary to immunosuppressive therapy leading to increased HCV RNA titres (Periera et al., 1995; Burstein & Rodby, 1993). In renal transplant recipients, HCV infection has been implicated in pathogenesis of acute glomerulopathy, de novo immune complex glomerulonephritis in allograft, and chronic allograft nephropathy (CAN) (Cosio et al., 1996; Roth et al., 1995; Ozdemir et al., 2006; Morales et al., 1997; Mahmoud et al., 2005). De novo membranoproliferative glomerulonephritis (MPGN), and de novo membranous glomerulonephritis (MGN), with or without mixed cryoglobulinemia are the most frequent glomerular patterns of injury seen in association with HCV infection in renal allografts. In 2001, one study reported the prevalence of de novo MPGN and MGN to be 45.4% and 18.2% in HCV positive transplant recipients as compared to 5.7% and 7.7% in HCV negative recipients (Cruzado et al., 2001). Subsequently, another study in 2006 reported the prevalence of de novo GN to be 34% in HCV infected recipients and only 6.6% in HCV negative recipients (Ozdemir et al., 2005). In general higher prevalence of autoimmune GN was associated with poor graft outcome, and even worse than de novo GN in HCV negative patients (Carbone et al., 2011).

Proteinuria is a common manifestation of kidney disease in HCV infected patients and renal biopsy is used to establish the diagnosis of glomerular injury, however currently it is impossible to determine HCV as the cause of glomerular damage based solely on morphologic assessment of renal biopsy. (Natov & Periera, 2012).

In 2005, Mahmoud et al reported a higher rate of CAN in HCV infected patients who did not receive interferon (IFN) therapy prior to renal transplant. Recent data also shows increased rate of graft failure due to CAN in HCV positive recipients than HCV negative (Scott et al., 2010). The Spanish Chronic Allograft Nephropathy Group analyzed 4304 renal transplant recipients with 587 of them being HCV positive over a period of 1990 to 2002. The study reported HCV infection to be associated with early proteinuria, lower renal function, de novo GN, chronic rejection, graft loss, and lower survival than HCV negative recipients (Morales et al., 2010). Another implication of HCV infection is its association with development of early graft dysfunction due to acute glomerular lesion. Examples of such lesions include acute transplant glomerulopathy, and de novo renal thrombotic microangiopathy (Cosio et al., 1996, Baid et al., 1995). Acute transplant glomerulopathy is mostly considered to be an atypical variant of acute cellular rejection and is also present more commonly in HCV positive recipients (Cosio et al., 1996a, 1996b).

3. Diagnosis

Detection of HCV infection is based primarily on the type of laboratory test used and its sensitivity and specificity. Any false positive tests will lead to unnecessary waste of precious potential organs for transplant (Natov & Periera, 2012). A large collaborative study was performed in United States that looked at the positive and negative predictive values of antibody screening tests. Eight organ procurement organizations representing different geographical regions studied 3078 cadaver organ donors. Using first generation enzyme linked immunosorbent assay ELISA1 anti-HCV test, the prevalence was found to be 5.1% (1.5-16.7%). Using the second generation ELISA2, the prevalence was 4.2%, with positive predictive value of 55% and negative predictive value of 100%. Some investigators have suggested the use of third generation ELISA3 tests to screen cadavers for HCV that because of its improved specificity showed only 3.7% prevalence. On the other hand, the prevalence of HCV RNA (ribonuclease acid) detection by Polymerase chain reaction (PCR) was only 2.4%. Although discarding all ELISA2 positive organs would eliminate transmission of HCV, there will be waste of 1.8% that will be discarded based on ELISA2 positivity while they are HCV RNA negative. However, it is currently not practical to test cadavers for HCV RNA status prior to organ procurement (Challine et al., 2004). The current practice in major centers is still to screen organ donors for antibodies against HCV. The serum aminotransferase levels are usually normal in uremic patients, and therefore are not considered reliable in determining disease activity and severity of fibrosis in this group. For clinically suspicious patients with elevated serum aminotransferase levels but negative antibody test, an HCV RNA assay with a detection limit of less than 50 IU/mL is recommended to rule out infection (Pawlotsky, 2002).

There is limited data on the impact of different HCV genotypes on survival after transplantation. Data reported by New England Organ Bank had relatively small number of patients and HCV genotype distribution to reach a conclusion (Natov et al., 1999).

Liver biopsy remains the gold standard for assessment of liver damage and fibrosis. Several scoring systems are used for assessment of hepatic fibrosis that use various criteria such as activity index and special stains for collagen deposition. Examples of these scoring systems include hepatic activity index (HAI), Knodell score and the Matavir system. Patients with HCV infection can have evidence of histologic liver disease in the absence of elevated transaminases and abnormal liver function tests. Therefore there may be merit in performing liver biopsy on all anti-HCV positive patients on transplant wait list. In patients with histologic evidence of liver disease, the decision to proceed or not with transplantation should be made with extreme caution as post-transplant immunosuppression may exacerbate liver disease (Zylerberg et al., 2002).

4. Clinical outcome with impact of HCV status before transplantation, and use of allografts from HCV positive donors

HCV has multiple distinct variants that are classified into six major types based on the viral genome sequence analysis. Each type consists of subtypes named in order of discovery such as a,b, c and so on, the subtypes may include individual isolates. Repeated infection or superinfection may occur in the same patient by the same or a different strain as HCV does

7

not provide immunity. Thus transplant recipients that are positive for HCV RNA may have the viral genotype of the donor, same genotype as present pretransplant or both individual genotypes. The impact of superinfection is not clear, however there is some evidence that HCV infection by one or multiple strains does not impact the survival negatively, at least in the short term (Natov et al., 1999; Natov & Periera, 2012; Ali et al., 1998).

The use of renal allografts from HCV positive donors to be transplanted in HCV infected recipients may offer some advantage (Figure 3) (Abbott et al., 2003). This approach is consistent with 2008 Kidney Disease: Improving Global Outcomes (KDIGO) Guideline recommendations (KDIGO, 2008). A survey was performed in United States on 245 transplant centers with response obtained from 147 centers. The data showed that 49% of these centers use HCV seropositive donors (Batiuk et al., 2002). Patients who are HCV positive before transplant have a significantly higher risk of developing posttransplant liver disease, mainly chronic hepatitis and its sequelae. An unusual serious form of liver involvement termed fibrosing cholestatic hepatitis has been reported in such patients. it is characterized by severe cholestasis, extensive fibrosis, and rapidly progressive liver failure, and is most likely related to acute infection under maximum immunosuppression (Toth et al., 1998; Delladetsima et al., 2006). Kidney transplant in HCV positive patients is associated with a 1.8-30.3 fold increase in serum viral titer most likely due to increased viral proliferation secondary to immunosuppressive therapy. However, this increase in viral titer may not be associated with increased risk of posttransplant liver disease, neither does it have any association with transaminase pattern or histologic severity of liver injury (Natov & Periera, 2012; Periera et al., 1995; Rpth et al., 1996).

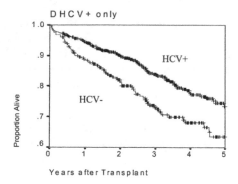

Figure 3. Kaplan-Meier plot of patient survival after renal transplantation, limited to patients who received a kidney positive for hepatitis C (DHCV+; n = 873) stratified by recipients who were HCV+ and HCV−. Reprinted from J Am Soc Nephol, 14, 2908-2918 (2003), Abbott K et al., Hepatitis C and Renal Transplantation in the Era of Modern Immunosuppression. With permission through Copyright Clearance Center

Mycophenolate mofetil and antithymocyte globulin are reported to increase HCV viremia while cyclosporine was found to have a suppressive effect on HCV replicon RNA level and HCV protein expression in cultured human hepatocytes (Figure 4) (Abbott et al., 2003; Rostaing et al., 2000; Geith, 2011; Misiani et al., 1994).

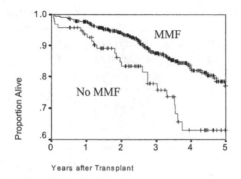

Figure 4. Kaplan-Meier plot of patient survival after renal transplantation, limited to patients who received a kidney positive for hepatitis C (DHCV+; n = 873) stratified by recipients who received mycophenolate mofetil (MMF) or those who did not (no MMF). Reprinted from J Am Soc Nephol, 14, 2908-2918 (2003), Abbott K et al., Hepatitis C and Renal Transplantation in the Era of Modern Immunosuppression. With permission through Copyright Clearance Center

Although there is solid data that shows increased risk of developing liver disease in HCV positive patients, there are conflicting reports and data regarding impact on survival. Some studies failed to show any difference in overall survival in transplant recipients that were HCV positive or negative. Other studies of pretransplant HCV positive recipients reported increased mortality rate mainly due to liver disease and sepsis with a 3.3 fold increased risk of death and 9.9 fold higher risk of mortality due to sepsis (Natov & Periera, 2012; Periera et al., 1995; Legendre et al., 1998). A 2005 meta-analysis on eight clinical trials involving a cohort of 6365 patients showed an increased relative risk of death in HCV positive patients (1.79) mainly due to liver cirrhosis and cancer. In addition the relative risk of allograft failure was 1.56 (Fabrizi et al., 2005).

Studies conducted in the 80s and 90s showed 35% of recipients who received allografts from HCV positive donors developed posttransplant liver disease, 50% became anti HCV positive after transplant, and 73% developed HCV viremia (Natov, 2002; Periera et al., 1994). The wide variation in the rate of transmission could be related to different prevalence among donors, difference in organ preservation and failure to test recipients in some centers. A large registry analysis in 2002 showed increased mortality in recipients of allografts from HCV positive donors regardless of the HCV status of the recipient (Bucci et al., 2002). Using the data from the Organ Procurement and Transplantation Network (OPTN), Maluf reported approximately 300 days shortening of wait time for HCV positive recipients receiving allografts from HCV positive donors compared with HCV negative recipients however there was significantly decreased graft and patient overall survival (Maluf et al., 2010). A larger analysis of the same data from OPTN was performed recently by Northup and colleagues in 2010 that included 19496 HCV positive recipients and 934 HCV positive donors. It showed the adjusted hazard ratio for death to be similar for HCV positive recipients of HCV positive donors and HCV positive recipients of HCV negative donors. The worst survival was seen in HCV negative recipients who received allografts from HCV positive donors (Northup et al., 2010).

In regards to superinfection, HCV genotype 1 is the most common genotype of HCV seen in Western countries and is notorious to be less responsive to antiviral therapy including Pegylated IFN and Ribavirin. Some authorities suggest that genotyping should be done routinely and genotype 1 renal allografts should not be used in recipients with other genotypes. However data is limited regarding this strategy (Carbone et al., 2011).

5. Treatment

In non-transplant setting, the combination therapy with interferon (IFN) and Ribavirin is the standard of care for treatment of initial as well as relapse of HCV infection. Clearance of Ribavirin is impaired in patients with renal dysfunction as the drug itself and its metabolites cannot be removed by Hemodialysis. Therefore, Ribavirin is not recommended in patients with creatinine clearance of less than 50mL/min. IFN therapy is however recommended in dialysis patients. The goal of pretranslant HCV treatment is to attempt to eradicate HCV before transplant subsequently leading to decrease in the risk of progression of HCV-associated liver disease, reduced risk of posttransplant renal dysfunction, and possible reduction in HCV disease progression. The optimal treatment of HCV in dialysis patients is regarded as IFN therapy but it is not known whether there is any added advantage on the use of pegylated IFN over nonpegylated standard IFN. Dialysis patients are not considered candidates of combination therapy owing to concerns regarding development of Ribavirin-induced anemia as the clearance of the drug is impaired in patients with renal dysfunction. A safer but less cost-effective approach is to use IFN therapy to treat HCV positive patients on dialysis who are potential transplant candidates. This strategy seems to have a beneficial effect on the course of liver disease posttransplant, shows higher rates of sustained biochemical and virological response, and seems to have reduced risk of HCV disease progression. At present data on relapse rate on HCV positive patients treated pretransplant is limited and controversial. 2008 KDIGO guidelines suggest HCV positive transplant candidates to be considered for IFN therapy before transplant. Ribavirin is not recommended because of its impaired clearance. Similar concerns apply to pegylated IFN because of its longer half-life and is also not recommended for pretransplant HCV therapy.

Posttransplant HCV treatment is generally not recommended. A major limitation to the use of IFN posttransplant is the potential of developing acute rejection. In addition to antiviral activity, IFN also has pleiotropic effects including antiproliferative and immunomodulatory functions. The National Institute of Health (NIH) Consensus Statement on management of HCV infection lists renal transplant as one of the contraindications to IFN therapy. Most authorities are in line with this approach because of the increased risk of acute rejection, high cost, limited efficacy, and significant side effects that are reported with IFN treatment after transplant. Treatment may be recommended in exceptional and life-threatening cases of HCV complications such as fibrosing cholestatic hepatitis, life-threatening vasculitis, recurrent and progressive HCV-associated glomerulopathy in the transplanted kidney, and advanced histologic stages of liver fibrosis.

2008 KDIGO guidelines recommend monotherapy with standard IFN only to be considered in HCV positive kidney transplant recipients (Terraut & Adey, 2007; Kim et al., 2011; Carbone et al., 2011; Natov & Periera, 2012. Data on efficacy of Ribavirin treatment alone after transplant is limited. Combination therapy is the most likely regimen to achieve a sustained virologic response (SVR), however Ribavirin dosage must be adjusted based on the renal function to minimize the complication of anemia.

Large scale, multicenter clinical trials are needed to determine the optimal treatment approach in these populations. New therapies may offer specific advantages and show decreased incidence of treatment-related side effects than the currently available drugs.

In addition SVR to antiviral therapy in patients with HCV associated renal disease has been associated with improvement in renal histology with reduced inflammation and immune deposits. Recently, five HCV positive renal transplant patients who developed type III cryoglobulinemic MPGN were successfully treated by Rituximab (anti-CD 20) chimeric monoclonal antibody (Basse et al., 2005, 2006).

Transplantation after adequate antiviral therapy followed by minimal immunosuppression can be a good option. Recently, Shah and colleagues evaluated graft function and graft as well as patient survival in retrospective analyses of 132 HCV-positive renal transplant patients who received tolerance induction protocol (TIP) with minimal immunosuppression and compared them with 79 controls transplanted using standard triple immunosuppression drugs. TIP consisted of 1 donor-specific transfusion, peripheral blood stem cell infusion, portal infusion of bone marrow, and target-specific irradiation. In the TIP group patient survival at 1, 5, and 10 years was 92.4%, 70.4%, and 63.7%, respectively, versus 75.6%, 71.7%, and 55.7% in the control group. The graft survival was 92.9%, 81.5%, and 79.1% versus 91.7%, 75.7%, and 67.7%, respectively. Rejection episodes were less frequent in the former group. Abnormal liver enzymes were seen in 22% patients in the TIP group versus 31% of the control group (Shah et al., 2011).

6. Conclusion

HCV infection is relatively common among patients with ESRD on dialysis and kidney transplant recipients. It is a major cause of morbidity and mortality among this group. When indicated, treatment with IFN and antiviral therapy should be commenced prior to kidney transplantation. The optimal treatment of transplant patients with HCV infection is not known. IFN is not recommended posttransplant because of potential risk of rejection. However there are some life threatening HCV related complications that would compel the use of IFN in a renal transplant recipient. In conclusion, Ribavirin is contraindicated in dialysis patients and alternative drugs are needed to enhance antiviral effects of IFN. For renal transplant recipients, Ribavirin can be used in combination with IFN in patients with restored renal function, however the risk of acute rejection with IFN therapy remains a serious concern. Alternative drugs are also needed with better safety and efficacy for treatment of HCV posttransplant. Despite the ongoing dilemma HCV positive renal transplant recipients have a better survival than HCV positive patients awaiting transplantation. Data shows strong evidence that use of allografts from HCV positive donors leads to reduced wait time for HCV positive recipients however there is conflicting data about graft and overall survival that needs to be further studied. In addition transplant of kidneys from HCV positive donors should be restricted to recipients with HCV viremia at the time of transplant.

Author details

A.A. Amir[1], R.A. Amir[2] and S.S. Sheikh[3]

1 Consultant Nephrologist, Dhahran Health Center, Saudi Aramco Medical Services Organization, Dhahran, Saudi Arabia

2 Dammam University, Dhahran, Saudi Arabia

3 Chief, Pathology and Laboratory Services, Dhahran Health Center, Saudi Aramco Medical Services Organization, Dhahran, Saudi Arabia

References

[1] Abbott, K, Bucci, J, Matsumoto, C, et al. Hepatitis C and renal transplantation in the era of modern immunosuppression. Journal of American Society of Nephrology, (2003). doi:ASN.0000090743.43034.72, 14, 2908-2918.

[2] Abbott, K. C, Lentine, K. L, Bucci, J. R, et al. The impact of transplantation with deceased donor hepatitis c-positive kidneys on survival in wait-listed long-term dialysis patients. Am J Transplant (2004).

[3] Abbott, K, Lentine, K, Bucci, J, et al. Impact of diabetes and hepatitis after kidney transplantation on patients who are affected by hepatitis C virus," Journal of the American Society of Nephrology, (2004). , 15(12), 3166-3174.

[4] Ali, M. K, Light, J. A, Barhyte, D. Y, et al. Donor hepatitis C virus status does not adversely affect short-term outcomes in HCV+ recipients in renal transplantation. Transplantation (1998).

[5] Alric, L. DiMartino V, Selves J, et al., "Long-term impact of renal transplantation on liver fibrosis during hepatitis C virus infection," Gastroenterology, (2002). , 123(5), 1494-1499.

[6] Baid, S, Pascual, M, Williams, W, et al. Renal thrombotic microangiopathy associated with anticardiolipin antibodies in hepatitis C virus-infected renal allograft recipients," Transplantation, (1995). , 59, 1676.

[7] Burstein, D. M, & Rodby, R. A. Membranoproliferative glomerulonephritis associated with hepatitis C virus infection. J Am Soc Nephrol (1993).

[8] Basse, G, Ribes, D, Kamar, N, Mehrenberger, M, Esposito, L, Guitard, J, Lavayssière, L, Oksman, F, Durand, D, Dur, D, & Rostaing, L. Rituximab therapy for de novo mixed cryoglobulinemia in renal transplant patients. Transplantation. (2005).

[9] Basse, G, Ribes, D, Kamar, N, Mehrenberger, M, Sallusto, F, Esposito, L, Guitard, J, Lavayssière, L, Oksman, F, Durand, D, & Rostaing, L. Rituximab therapy for mixed cryoglobulinemia in seven renal transplant patients. Transplant Proc. (2006).

[10] Batiuk, T. D, Bodziak, K. A, & Goldman, M. Infectious disease prophylaxis in renal transplant patients: a survey of US transplant centers. Clin Transplant (2002).

[11] Bucci, J, Matsumoto, C, Swanson, S, Agodoa, L, Holtzmuller, K, & Abbott, K. Donor hepatitis C seropositivity: clinical correlates and effect on early graft and patient survival in adult cadaveric kidney transplantation," Journal of the American Society of Nephrology, (2002). , 13(12), 2974-2982.

[12] Carbone, M, Cockwell, P, & Neuberger, J. Hepatitis c and kidney transplantation. *International journal of nephrology, 2011*(593291), 1-17. doi:

[13] "NIH consensus statement on management of hepatitis C: (2002). NIH Consens State Sci Statements, , 19(3), 1-46.

[14] Challine, D, Pellegrin, B, Bouvier-alias, M, et al. HIV and hepatitis C virus RNA in seronegative organ and tissue donors, Lancet (2004).

[15] Cosio, G, Sedmak, D. D, Henry, M. L, et al. The high prevalence of severe early posttransplant renal allograft pathology inhepatitis C positive recipients," Transplantation, (1996). , 62(8), 1054-1059.

[16] Cosio, F. G, Roche, Z, Agarwal, A, et al. Prevalence of hepatitis C in patients with idiopathic glomerulopathies in native and transplant kidneys. Am J Kidney Dis (1996).

[17] Cosio, F. G, Sedmak, D. D, Henry, M. L, et al. The high prevalence of severe early post-transplant renal allograft pathology in hepatitis C positive recipients. Transplantation (1996).

[18] Cruzado, J, Carrera, M, Torras, J, & Griny, J ′ o. Hepatitis C virus infection and de novo glomerular lesions in renal allografts," American Journal of Transplantation, (2001). , 1(2), 171-178.

[19] Delladetsima, I, Psichogiou, M, Sypsa, V, et al. The course of hepatitis C virus infection in pretransplantation antihepatitis C virus-negative renal transplant recipients: a retrospective follow-up study," American Journal of Kidney Diseases, (2006). , 47(2), 309-316.

[20] Fabrizi, F, Poordad, F, & Martin, P. Hepatitis C infection and the patient with end-stage renal disease," Hepatology, (2002). , 36(1), 3-10.

[21] Fabrizi, F, Martin, P, Dixit, V, Bunnapradist, S, & Dulai, G. Meta-analysis: effect of hepatitis C virus infection on mortality in dialysis," Alimentary Pharmacology and Therapeutics,(2004). , 20(11-12), 1271-1277.

[22] Fabrizi, F, Martin, P, Dixit, V, Bunnapradist, S, & Dulai, G. Hepatitis C virus antibody status and survival after renal transplantation: meta-analysis of observational studies," American Journal of Transplantation, (2005). , 5(6), 1452-1461.

[23] Fabrizi, F, Takkouche, B, Lunghi, G, Dixit, V, Messa, P, & Martin, P. The impact of hepatitis C virus infection on survival in dialysis patients: meta-analysis of observational studies," Journal of Viral Hepatitis, (2007). , 14(10), 697-703.

[24] Finelli, L, Miller, J, Tokars, J, & Arduino, M. National surveillance of dialysis-associated diseases in the United States, 2002," Seminars in Dialysis, (2005). , 18(1), 52-61.

[25] Fissell, R, Bragg-gresham, J, Woods, J, et al. Patterns of hepatitis C prevalence and seroconversion in hemodialysis units from three continents: the DOOPS," Kidney International, (2004). , 65(6), 2335-2342.

[26] Gheith, O. Dilemma of HCV infection in renal transplant recipients". International Journal of Nephrology 2011: 471214, (2011). doi:

[27] Goodkin, D, Bragg-gresham, J, Koenig, K, et al. Association of comorbid conditions and mortality in hemodialysis patients in Europe, Japan, and the United States: the dialysis outcomes and practice patterns study (DOPPS)," Journal of the American Society of Nephrology, (2003). , 14(12), 3270-3277.

[28] Gürsoy, M, Köksal, R, Karavelioglu, D, Colak, T, Gür, G, Ozdemir, N, Boyacioglu, S, & Bilgin, N. Pretransplantation alpha-interferon therapy and the effect of hepatitis C virus infection on kidney allograft recipients. Transplant Proc. (2000).

[29] Jadoul, M, Poignet, J, Geddes, C, et al. The changing epidemiology of hepatitis C virus infection in haemodialysis: European multicentre study," Nephrology Dialysis Transplantation, (2004). , 19(4), 904-909.

[30] Kidney disease: improving global outcome (KDIGO)KDIGO clinical practice guidelines for the prevention, diagnosis, evaluation, and treatment of hepatitis C in chronic kidney disease. Kidney Int Suppl (2008). suppl 109):s1

[31] KDIGO clinical practice guidelines for the preventiondiagnosis, evaluation, and treatment of hepatitis C in chronic kidney disease. Kidney Int (2008). Suppl 109):S1.

[32] Kim, E, Ko, H, & Yoshida, E. (2011). Treatment issues surrounding hepatitis c in renal transplantation: A review. Annals of hepatology, 10(1), 5-14.

[33] Knoll, G. A, Tankersley, M. R, Lee, J. Y, et al. The impact of renal transplantation on survival in hepatitis C-positive end-stage renal disease patients. Am J Kidney Dis (1997).

[34] Legendre, C, & Garrigue, V. Le Bihan C, et al. Harmful long-term impact of hepatitis C virus infection in kidney transplant recipients. Transplantation (1998).

[35] Mahmoud, I, Sobh, M, Habashi, A, et al. Interferon therapy in hemodialysis patients with chronic hepatitis C: study of tolerance, efficacy and post-transplantation course," Nephron Clinical Practice, (2005). , 100(4), c133-c139.

[36] Maluf, D. G, Fisher, R. A, King, A. L, et al. Hepatitis C virus infection and kidney transplantation: predictors of patient and graft survival. Transplantation (2007).

[37] Maluf, D, Archer, K, & Mas, V. Kidney grafts from HCV-positive donors: advantages and disadvantages," Transplantation Proceedings, (2010). , 42(7), 2436-2446.

[38] Mendez, R, Shahawy, M, Obispo, E, et al. Four years follow up of hepatitis C positive kidneys into hepatitis C negative recipients- Prospective study. J Am Soc Nephrol (1995).

[39] Misiani, R, Bellavita, P, Fenili, D, Vicari, O, Marchesi, D, Sironi, P. L, Zilio, P, Vernocchi, A, & Massazza, M. Venderamin G: Interferon alfa-2a therapy in cryoglobulinenia associated with hepatitis C virus. N Engl J Med , 330, 751-756.

[40] Morales, J, Pascual-capdevila, J, Campistol, J, et al. Membranous glomerulonephritis associated with hepatitis C virus infection in renal transplant patients," Transplantation, (1997). , 63(11), 1634-1639.

[41] Morales, J. Marc'en R, Andres A, et al., "Renal transplantation in patients with hepatitis C virus antibody. A long national experience," NDT Plus, supplement 2, (2010). , 3, ii41-ii46.

[42] Natov, S. Transmission of viral hepatitis by kidney transplantation:donor evaluation and transplant policies (part 1:hepatitis B virus)," Transplant Infectious Disease, (2002). , 4(3), 124-131.

[43] Natov, S. N, Lau, J. Y, Ruthazer, R, et al. Hepatitis C virus genotype does not affect patient survival among renal transplant candidates. The New England Organ Bank Hepatitis C Study Group. Kidney Int (1999).

[44] Natov, S, & Pereira, B. (2012). Hepatitis c virus infection and renal translpantation. In D. Brennan & A. Sheridan (Eds.), Retrieved from http://www.uptodate.com/contents/hepatitis-c-virus-infection-and-renal-transplantation

[45] Natov, S, & Pereira, B. (2012). Renal disease associated with hepatitis c virus after renal transplantation. In D. Brennan, M. Hirsch & A. Sheridan (Eds.), Retrieved from http://www.uptodate.com/contents/renal-disease-associated-with-hepatitis-c-virus-after-renal-tranplantation

[46] Northup, P, Argo, C, Nguyen, D, et al. Liver allografts from hepatitis c positive donors can offer good outcomes in hepatitis C positive recipients: a us national transplant registry analysis," Transplant International, (2010). , 23(10), 1038-1044.

[47] Ozdemir, B, Ozdemir, F, Sezer, S, Colak, T, & Haberal, M. De novo glomerulonephritis in renal allografts with hepatitis C virus infection," Transplantation Proceedings, (2006)., 38(2), 492-495.

[48] Pawlotsky JM: Molecular diagnosis of viral hepatitis Gstroenterology 122: 1554-1568, (2002).

[49] Pedroso, S, Martins, L, Fonseca, I, et al. Impact of Hepatitis C virus on renal transplantation: Association with poor survival. Transplantation Proceedings, (2006). doi:j.transproceed.2006.06.065, 38, 1890-1894.

[50] Periera, B. J, Milford, E. L, Kirkman, R. L, & Levey, A. S. Transmission of hepatitis C virus by organ transplantation. N Engl J Med (1991).

[51] Periera, B. J, Wright, T. L, Schmid, C. H, et al. Screening and confirmatory testing of cadaver organ donors for hepatitis C virus infection: a U.S. National Collaborative Study, Kidney Int (1994).

[52] Periera, B, Wright, T, Schmid, C, et al. Screening and confirmatory testing of cadaver organ donors for hepatitis C virus infection: a U.S. national collaborative study," Kidney International, (1994)., 46(3), 886-892.

[53] Periera, B. J, Wright, T. L, Schmid, C. H, & Levey, A. S. The impact of pretransplantation hepatitis C infection on the outcome of renal transplantation. Transplantation (1995).

[54] Periera, B. J, Wright, T. L, Schmid, C. H, & Levey, A. S. Transmission of hepatitis C transmission by organ transplantation. The New England Organ Bank Hepatitis C Study Group. Lancet (1995).

[55] Pereira, B, & Levey, A. Hepatitis C virus infection in dialysis and renal transplantation," Kidney International, (1997)., 51(4), 981-999.

[56] Pereira, B. J, Natov, S. N, Bouthot, B. A, et al. Effects of hepatitis C infection and renal transplantation on survival in end-stage renal disease. The New England Organ Bank Hepatitis C Study Group. Kidney Int (1998).

[57] Pirsch, J, Heisey, D, & Allesandro, D. A, et al. Transplantation of hepatitis C (HCV) kidneys: Defining the risks (abstract). 14th Annual Meeting of the American Society of Transplant Physicians, Chicago, May 14-17, (1995)., 98.

[58] Poynard, T, Ratziu, V, Charlotte, F, Goodman, Z, Mchutchison, J, & Albrecht, J. Rates and risk factors of liver fibrosis progression in patients with chronic hepatitis C," Journal of Hepatology, (2001)., 34(5), 730-739.

[59] Rostaing, L, Izopet, J, Sandres, K, et al. Changes in hepatitis C virus RNA viremia concentrations in long-term renal transplant patients after introduction of Mycophenolate mofetil. Transplantation (2000).

[60] Roth, D, Cirocco, R, Zucker, K, et al. De novo membranoproliferative glomerulo-
    nephritis in hepatitis C virus infected renal allograft recipients," Transplantation,
    (1995). , 59(12), 1676-1682.

[61] Roth, D, Zucker, K, Cirocco, R, et al. A prospective study of hepatitis C virus infec-
    tion in renal allograft recipients. Transplantation (1996).

[62] Shah, P, Vanikar, A, Gumber, M, Patel, H, Kute, V, Godara, S, & Trivedi, H. (2011).
    Renal transplantation in hepatitis c positive patients: A single centre experience.
    Journal of transplantation, doi:, 2011, 1-5.

[63] Scott, D, Wong, J, Spicer, T, et al. Adverse impact of hepatitis C virus infection on re-
    nal replacement therapy and renal transplant patients in Australia and New Zea-
    land," Transplantation, (2010). , 90(11), 1165-1171.

[64] Terrault, N, & Adey, D. (2007). The kidney transplant recipient with hepatitis c infec-
    tion pre- and posttransplantation treatment. American society of nephrology,
    doi:CJN.02930806, 2, 563-575.

[65] Toth, C. M, Pascual, M, Chung, R. T, et al. Hepatitis C virus-associated fibrosing cho-
    lestatic hepatitis after renal transplantation: response to interferon-alpha therapy.
    Transplantation (1998).

[66] Watashi, K, Hijikata, M, Hosaka, M, et al. Cyclosporin A suppresses replication of
    hepatitis C virus genome in cultured hepatocytes. Hepatology (2003).

[67] Zylberberg, H, Nalpas, B, Carnot, F, et al. Severe evolution of chronic hepatitis C in
    renal transplantation: a case control study. Nephrol Dial Transplant (2002).

[68] Zylberberg, H, Nalpas, B, Carnot, F, et al. Severe evolution of chronic hepatitis C in
    renal transplantation: a case control study," Nephrology Dialysis Transplantation,
    (2002). , 17(1), 129-133

Comparison of Renal Transplantation Outcomes in Patients After Peritoneal Dialysis and Hemodialysis – A Case Control Study and Literature Review

Thomas Rath and Stephan Ziefle

Additional information is available at the end of the chapter

1. Introduction

For patients with end-stage renal disease renal transplantation is the treatment of choice. However, there is still some controversy if mortality rate after renal transplantation is affected by the chosen dialysis modality.

It is widely accepted, that in terms of survival hemodialysis (HD) and peritoneal dialysis (PD) are comparable. Especially in PD-patients with preserved residual renal function, control of hypertension is achieved more easily, whereas patients with diabetes mellitus do better on HD. In general, quality of life for patients is assumed to be better with PD than with HD [1].

In a cost-modeling strategy, incorporating quality of life and social perspective aspects in Scandinavia, it was shown, that the cost per quality-adjusted life year for PD was lower compared to HD in all analyzed age groups, whereas mean survival and frequency of transplantation did not differ [2].

Despite technological advance, only 15 % of the world dialysis population is managed by PD. Therefore, a "integrated approach" suggests starting PD in alarge percentage of patients, especially when renal transplantation is expected in the next 2 or 3 years after initiation of dialysis [3].

A very interesting point became obvious when analyzing data obtained from the Dialysis Morbidity and Mortality Study Wave 2, a national random sample of more than 4000 new dialysis patients in the USA enrolled during 1996 and 1997 and followed up until 2001. There, it was shown, that transplantation rates were significantly higher for patients reporting the greatest contribution to modality selection. These results support the association of patient autonomy with transplantation and survival, probably in favor for patients actively choosing PD as their dialysis modality [4]. Also, a small Japanese single center study in 42 patients analyzed the effect of dialysis modality on rate of kidney transplantation from living donors and transplant outcome. There were no differences between the two modalities prior to transplantation in the graft survival rate, incidence of acute rejection, and complications before and after transplantation.However, The transfer rate from PD to transplantation was significantly (p = 0.0036) higher (4.7%) than that of HD (1.9%). Probably reflecting better cooperation between with the patients, their family and the provision of relevant information by nephrologists during PD [5].

2. Mortality on PD and HD

Although in 2005 the European Best Practice Guidelines for Peritoneal Dialysis conclude, on the basis of the available data, that peritoneal dialysis is a good treatment prior to renal transplantation there are contradictory survival rates reported in the literature for patients either on HD or on PD[6].

In 1995, data from the US Renal Data Systems from more than 170,000 patients showed, thatprevalent patients treated with PD had a 19% higher adjusted mortality risk (p< 0.001) than those treated with HD [7].

In a comparable analysis obtained from the Canadian Organ Replacement Register, using data from 11,970 ESRD patientswho initiated treatment between 1990 and 1994 and were followed-up for a maximum of 5 years was themortality rate ratio for CAPD/CCPD relative to hemodialysis, as estimated by Poisson regression, was 0.73. There, the increased mortality on hemodialysis compared with CAPD/CCPD was concentrated in the first 2 years of follow-up and was detectable in all subgroups defined by age and diabetes status [8].

In contrast, a study comparing two year mortality rates of patients on the waiting list for renal transplantation to a historical prospective cohort of more than 12000 PD and HD patients disclosed, that especially for patients with a body mass index (BMI) of>= 26 mortality was increased with PD as dialysis modality [9].

Nevertheless, in a cohort of more than 3000 non-diabetic patients starting dialysis there was no difference in survival for patients treated either with PD or HD [10].

Also, in the well-known, prospective Netherlands Cooperative Study on the Adequacy of Dialysis (NECOSAD) adjusted mortality rates between HD and PD patients were similar for the first two years. Thereafter, an increase in mortality especially in patients >= 60 years was detected [11].

Comparable results were seen in a prospective multicenter cohort study in 1041 patients (767 HD, 274 PD). There, the risk of mortality was equal in both groups for the first year with an increase in the second year. In addition, 25% of PD but only 5% of the HD patients switched their type of dialysis modality [12].

3. Renal transplantation in PD–patients – first experience

The first experience about the use of peritoneal dialysis in patients waiting for renal transplantation were published in some very early reports describing the feasibility of PD for patients awaiting renal transplantation[13-15]. Also in a small series of 15 patients the experience with renal transplantation in PD-patients was reported. Despite the fact, that some of the PD patients had peritonitis at the time of transplantation, no differences in graft survival were shown [16].

Similar results were published in an early study with a group of 44 patients, showing comparable results for patients with PD compared to HD patients[17].

Also, a small study in 9 PD patients reported significantly greater and longer wound drainage in PD patients. However, the incidence of acute rejection episodes, delayed graft function, graft arterial thrombosis and graft function recovery was not different [18].

4. PD versus HD and survival after renal transplantation

In a retrospective analysis of 61 PD and 159 HD patients there were no differences in survival of patients or grafts between the two treatment groups. One year after transplantation the percentages of survivors who had received continuous ambulatory peritoneal dialysis and hemodialysis were 88% and 91% respectively, and overall graft survival was 66% and 72%, respectively [19]. Similar results were reported from 42 PD patients, either treated with CAPD for more than 26 weeks or less than 26 weeks in comparison with 55 HD patients, irrespectively if treated with azathioprine + prednisolone or cyclosporine + prednisolone [20]. A retrospective analysis of 389 patients transplanted between Juli,1974, and July 1985, also evaluated the effect of dialysis modality on transplantation and mortality rates. By correcting for the influence of different variables and using time-dependent treatment co-variables, the bias adjusted estimates of the relative risk of death did not differ significantly from one another [21]. A cohort analysis of 500 first renal transplant recipients (241 on CAPD, 259 on HD) showed identical graft and patient survival after five years. However in 37 PD patients post-transplant peritoneal dialysis was necessary, while 10 patients developed peritonitis [22].

In 54 patients with renal transplantation after PD compared to 48 patients after HD with an immunosuppressive regimen consisting of prednisolone, azathioprine and cyclosporine there no significant difference in patient mortality and survival or graft survival between the groups. The incidences of infections were also similar in the two groups [23].

5. PD and complications after renal transplantation

There is some concern with respect for the risk of infections, especially peritonitis caused by the peritoneal catheter in PD patients. In a retrospective single center analysis the experience with 18 renal transplantations in 16 PD patients was reported. In two cases cultures of the peritoneal catheter removed a few days after successful transplantation were positive. Nevertheless, with adequate antibiotic treatment none of the patients ever developed clinical peritonitis [24].

A cohort analysis of 500 first renal transplant recipients (241 on CAPD, 259 on HD) showed identical graft and patient survival after five years. However, 10 PD patients developed peritonitis [21]. Also, in a series of 100 patients undergoing simultaneous pancreas-kidney (SPK) transplantation (25 PD patients, 75 HD patients) frequency of abdominal infections, one year pancreas-graft survival rates, acute rejection episodes, kidney graft survival rates, or length of hospital stay did not differ between the two groups[25].

The question of peritonitis in peritoneal dialysis patients after renal transplantation was also addressed by a retrospective, single center study of 232 PD patients. In total, 30 peritonitis episodes with predominantly Staphylococcus aureus (10/30) or gram-negative bacteria (12/30) were observed. Risk factors associated with post-transplant peritonitis were the total number of peritonitis episodes, previous peritonitis with S. aureus bacteria, male sex, technical surgical problems at the time of transplantation, more than two rejection episodes, permanent graft non-function, and urinary leakage [26].

Comparable results are reported in a two-center study on post-transplant PD-related complications in 137 PD patients. There, only in a minority of the patients (n=19) PD-catheters were removed on the time of transplantation. In the remaining 118 patients the peritonitis rate was 7% [27].

In the European Best Practice Guidelines for Peritoneal Dialysis it is recommended to remove the catheter early after transplantation, nevertheless the catheter could be left in situ for 3–4 months despite a functioning graft. The guidelines also state, that peritonitis and exit site infections in transplanted patients should be treated using the ISPD guidelines 6.

In the last years the problem of post-transplant diabetes mellitus (PTDM) has gained more attention. A single center study reports on the occurrence of PTDM in 72 renal transplant recipients. In univariate analysis, the factors associated with the elevated risk of PTDM appearance were treatment by PD, older recipient age, positive family history of diabetes, hypertensive nephropathy as end-stage renal disease cause, higher body mass index at transplantation, and the graft from an older donor [28].

PD may be associated with an increased risk for graft thrombosis. At least, a single center experience revealed that in 915 consecutive renal transplantations CAPD was associated with a growing frequency of renal allograft thrombosis (7.3% vs. 3.6 %, p<0.02). No differences in transplant characteristics, including hemodynamics, hematological parameters, immunosuppressive therapy, graft anatomy and preservation, were observed between the cases with graft thrombosis and a matched control group of 88 patients [29].

After renal allograft failure, patients may chose PD as their primary treatment option again. For this situation, it was shown, that after a failed renal transplantation PD-patients are prone to greater risk of death compared to PD-patients never transplanted. In addition, time to first peritonitis, subsequent episodes of peritonitis, catheter change, or transfer to hemodialysis occurred at a much faster rate in patients with a failed transplant [30].

For patients returning to PD after graft failure, there may be a survival advantage in maintaining them on long-term immunosuppressive therapy. At least, a decision analytic model comparing the use of immunosuppression after transplant failure and return to peritoneal dialysis with immunosuppressive withdrawal, lead the authors to conclude, that there may be a survival advantage in maintaining patients on long-term immunosuppression [31].

6. PD and the occurrence of delayed graft function after renal transplantation

It is well known, that delayed graft function (DGF) and acute renal failure (ARF) after renal transplantation negatively influence short- and long-term graft outcome, therefore it is of interest to know if peritoneal dialysis affects occurrence or severity of DGF after renal transplantation.

A study in 250 patients (70 PD, 180 HD) evaluated the influence of dialysis modality on transplant outcomes. Among HD patients, 16% displayed DGF, versus 12% of PD patients. Multivariate analysis showed that factors affecting DGF were mode of dialysis, serum concentrations of parathyroid hormone and C-Reactive-Protein, and hemoglobin levels. Also after 3 and 5 years follow-up, PD patients showed fewer graft failures than HD patients (14% vs. 20%; and 17% vs. 28%[32].

In an analysis of 92 PD patients and 587 HD patients there was higher immediate graft function, less delayed graft function and less patients with never functioning grafts in the PD group. The groups were comparable except for a higher prevalence of diabetes ($p < 0.05$) and a shorter time on dialysis ($p < 0.01$) in PD patients [33].

A retrospective study in 40 PD and 79 HD patients receiving their first renal transplant analyzed the occurrence and frequency of DGF and acute renal failure. Both, DGF and ARF were observed less in the PD group than in the HD group. In a multivariate model, the authors could show that PD as pre-transplantation modality favorably modified the relative risk of developing DGF and ARF after renal transplantation[34]. A single center analysis in more than 650 patients (92 PD, 587 HD) reports a higher rate of DGF in HD patients (39.5% vs. 22.5%) and a higher rate of never functioning grafts in HD patients compared to PD patients (14% vs. 9%). When potential risk factors for DGF were compared, no relevant differences could be found [33].

Also for PD patients on automated peritoneal dialysis (APD), a retrospective matched-pairs study with 67 APD-patients showed favorable effects for PD on initial graft function (patients with a creatinine clearance below 10 ml/min 6 days after surgery) after post-mortem renal transplantation [35].

A recent retrospective single center analysis in 38 PD and 268 HD patients describes a higher incidence of DGF and primary allograft failure for HD patients, but was no difference in acute rejection episodes, long-term survivals, or renal function [36].

A case control study the incidence of DGF, defined as necessity to perform dialysis after transplantation, was analyzed in 117 PD and HD patients with a follow-up of 6 months. When matching the patients for age, sex, HLA compatibility PD-patients developed less DGF (23.1%) than HD patients (50.4%). In addition the decline of creatinine levels after transplantation was faster in PD patients. However, PD patients developed more acute rejection episodes, than HD patients, but creatinine levels after 6 weeks and 6 months were not different between the groups [37].

Besides a bundle of published single center experiences with renal transplantation in PD patients we do have at least two registry studies reporting on the effect of pre-transplant dialysis modality on renal transplant results.

Data from the United Network of Organ Sharing on all cadaveric graft recipients who were dialysis-dependent at the time of transplantation were analyzed with respect to different outcomes in the immediate post-transplant period for HD or PD patients. In total more than 9000 patients were evaluated, showing that PD patients were on dialysis for a shorter period of time, were more likely to be white, had a better HLA match, and had a lower PRA. After adjusting for comorbidities, the odds of oliguria were 1.60 times higher in black HD patients compared with PD patients and 1.29 times higher in white HD patients. Also, the odds of requiring dialysis in the first week were 1.56 times higher in black HD patients versus PD patients and 1.40 times higher in white HD patients. The rate of acute rejection was similar during the first hospitalization. Therefore, the authors suggest that there may be an association between hemodialysis and delayed graft function assuming that differences in biocompatibility between the two modalities could potentially be responsible [38].

A large retrospective analysis compared transplantation rates in PD and HD and outcomes after transplantation in more than 22000 patients from the years 1995 to 1998 in a US cohort. PD patients were more likely to be transplanted and their death censored graft failure was higher. However, mortality and overall graft failure were not different. Interestingly, the risk for early graft failure was higher for PD patients despite DGF was less common [39].

7. Own experience with PD and renal transplantation

Because of the in part contradictory data published in the literature we analyzed our own population of renal transplant recipients with the means of a retrospective case control study. Therefore, we chose 50 consecutive peritoneal dialysis patients transplanted since 1999. For match-pair-analysis, and as control group we selected the next hemodialysis patient subsequently transplanted after each PD patient. Follow-up data were available with a maximum of ten years after transplantation.

Kruskal-Wallis Test and Chi-Square-Test were calculated, with assuming a $p<0.05$ as significant, for statistical purposes.

The PD-group consisted out of 28 male and 22 female patients with a mean age of 48.7 +/- 11.5 years (HD: 31 m, 19 w, 49,8 +/-13, p=n.s.) quite reflecting the German dialysis population. With respect to time on renal replacement therapy, cytomegalo-virus-status, HLA-mismatch, proportion of living donors, age, sex and initial immunosuppression there were no differences between the groups.

Although, during follow up more less PD-patients (n=3) than HD-patients (n=8) died, this difference did not reach statistical significance. With respect to graft failure, transplant loss (n=18) occurred significantly more in HD patients (n=13) than in PD patients (n=5). Nevertheless, mean serum-creatinine after 1, 2 and 5 years was not significant different between the groups. Also, delayed graft function was reported in only 4 PD patients compared to 10 HD patients (p<0.05).

To summarize, in our retrospective match-pair analysis patients on PD before renal transplantation developed less delayed graft function and had less graft loss during follow-up than patients on HD before transplantation.

8. Conclusion

Peritoneal dialysis (PD) is an established method of renal replacement therapy. PD and hemodialysis (HD) seem to be equivalent for long-term survival of the patients. Nevertheless, there is a beneficial effect of PD on patient survival after initiation of dialysis therapy. Probably, better preservation of residual renal function in PD patients compared to HD patients may be responsible for this effect.

Renal transplantation is the best treatment option for patients with endstage renal disease. The potential risk of infectious complications in PD patients after renal transplantation is attributed to the remaining PD catheter. However, this risk seems to be low and without effect on graft survival. For patients on HD a higher percentage of delayed graft function after renal transplantation is constantly reported in the literature. Nevertheless, long time patient and graft survival are not different between both treatment modalities.

Our own long-time clinical experience is congruent with the published literature and proves that peritoneal dialysis is a valuable treatment option for patients with end stage renal disease waiting for renal transplantation.

Author details

Thomas Rath* and Stephan Ziefle

*Address all correspondence to: trath@westpfalz-klinikum.de

Department of Nephrology and Transplantation Medicine, Westpfalz-Klinikum GmbH, Kaiserslautern, Germany

References

[1] Alloatti S, Manes M, Paternoster G, et al. Peritoneal dialysis compared with hemodialysis in the treatment of end-stage renal disease. J Nephrol 2000;13:331-42

[2] Sennfalt K, Magnusson M, Carlsson P. Comparison of hemodialysis and peritoneal dialysis--a cost-utility analysis. Perit Dial Int 2002;22:39-47

[3] Gradaus F, Ivens K, Peters AJ, et al. Angiographic progression of coronary artery disease in patients with end-stage renal disease. Nephrol Dial Transplant 2001;16:1198-202

[4] Stack AG, Martin DR. Association of patient autonomy with increased transplantation and survival among new dialysis patients in the United States. Am J Kidney Dis 2005;45:730-42

[5] Mitome J, Yamamoto H, Kato N, et al. [Dialysis as bridge therapy for renal transplantation: single center experience, a comparison of hemodialysis and continuous ambulatory peritoneal dialysis]. Nippon Jinzo Gakkai Shi 2005;47:813-20

[6] Dombros N, Dratwa M, Feriani M, et al. European best practice guidelines for peritoneal dialysis. 9 PD and transplantation. Nephrol Dial Transplant 2005;20 Suppl 9:ix34-ix35

[7] Bloembergen WE, Port FK, Mauger EA, Wolfe RA. A comparison of mortality between patients treated with hemodialysis and peritoneal dialysis. J Am Soc Nephrol 1995;6:177-83

[8] Fenton SS, Schaubel DE, Desmeules M, et al. Hemodialysis versus peritoneal dialysis: a comparison of adjusted mortality rates. Am J Kidney Dis 1997;30:334-42: published online , doi:S0272638697001686 [pii]

[9] Inrig JK, Sun JL, Yang Q, et al. Mortality by dialysis modality among patients who have end-stage renal disease and are awaiting renal transplantation. Clin J Am Soc Nephrol 2006;1:774-9

[10] Traynor JP, Thomson PC, Simpson K, et al. Comparison of patient survival in non-diabetic transplant-listed patients initially treated with haemodialysis or peritoneal dialysis. Nephrol Dial Transplant 2011;26:245-52: published online , doi:gfq361 [pii]; 10.1093/ndt/gfq361 [doi]

[11] Termorshuizen F, Korevaar JC, Dekker FW, et al. Hemodialysis and peritoneal dialysis: comparison of adjusted mortality rates according to the duration of dialysis: analysis of The Netherlands Cooperative Study on the Adequacy of Dialysis 2. J Am Soc Nephrol 2003;14:2851-60

[12] Jaar BG, Coresh J, Plantinga LC, et al. Comparing the risk for death with peritoneal dialysis and hemodialysis in a national cohort of patients with chronic kidney disease. Ann Intern Med 2005;143:174-83: published online , doi:143/3/174 [pii]

[13] Goldsmith Ei, Whitsell JC, Skelley K, Lubash Gd. Repeated peritoneal dialysis in preparation for renal transplantation. Surg Gynecol Obstet 1965;121:42-6

[14] Brunner FP, Scheitlin W. [Experiences with peritoneal dialysis in the preparation for kidney transplantation]. Z Gesamte Exp Med 1967;143:358-61

[15] Cohen SL, Percival A. Prolonged peritoneal dialysis in patients awaiting renal transplantation. Br Med J 1968;1:409-13

[16] Gokal R, Ramos JM, Veitch P, et al. Renal transplantation in patients on continuous ambulatory peritoneal dialysis. Proc Eur Dial Transplant Assoc 1981;18:222-7

[17] Diaz-Buxo JA, Walker PJ, Burgess WP, et al. The influence of peritoneal dialysis on the outcome of transplantation. Int J Artif Organs 1986;9:359-62

[18] Hrvacevic R, Maksic D, Aleksic S, et al. [Outcome of kidney transplantation in patients on peritoneal dialysis]. Vojnosanit Pregl 2001;58:471-4

[19] Donnelly PK, Lennard TW, Proud G, et al. Continuous ambulatory peritoneal dialysis and renal transplantation: a five year experience. Br Med J (Clin Res Ed) 1985;291:1001-4

[20] Evangelista JB, Jr., Bennett-Jones D, Cameron JS, et al. Renal transplantation in patients treated with haemodialysis and short term and long term continuous ambulatory peritoneal dialysis. Br Med J (Clin Res Ed) 1985;291:1004-7

[21] Burton PR, Walls J. Selection-adjusted comparison of life-expectancy of patients on continuous ambulatory peritoneal dialysis, haemodialysis, and renal transplantation. Lancet 1987;1:1115-9

[22] O'Donoghue D, Manos J, Pearson R, et al. Continuous ambulatory peritoneal dialysis and renal transplantation: a ten-year experience in a single center. Perit Dial Int 1992;12:242, 245-2, 249

[23] Kang Z, Fang G, Chen W. A comparative study of the outcome of renal transplantation in peritoneal dialysis and hemodialysis patients. Chin Med Sci J 1992;7:49-52

[24] Steinmuller D, Novick A, Braun W, et al. Renal transplantation of patients on chronic peritoneal dialysis. Am J Kidney Dis 1984;3:436-9

[25] Padillo-Ruiz J, Arjona-Sanchez A, Munoz-Casares C, et al. Impact of peritoneal dialysis versus hemodialysis on incidence of intra-abdominal infection after simultaneous pancreas-kidney transplant. World J Surg 2010;34:1684-8: published online , doi: 10.1007/s00268-010-0527-z [doi]

[26] Bakir N, Surachno S, Sluiter WJ, Struijk DG. Peritonitis in peritoneal dialysis patients after renal transplantation. Nephrol Dial Transplant 1998;13:3178-83

[27] Warren J, Jones E, Sener A, et al. Should peritoneal dialysis catheters be removed at the time of kidney transplantation? Can Urol Assoc J 2012;6:376-8: published online , doi:cuaj.12112 [pii];10.5489/cuaj.12112 [doi]

[28] Madziarska K, Weyde W, Krajewska M, et al. The increased risk of post-transplant diabetes mellitus in peritoneal dialysis-treated kidney allograft recipients. Nephrol Dial Transplant 2011;26:1396-401: published online , doi:gfq568 [pii];10.1093/ndt/gfq568 [doi]

[29] van der Vliet JA, Barendregt WB, Hoitsma AJ, Buskens FG. Increased incidence of renal allograft thrombosis after continuous ambulatory peritoneal dialysis. Clin Transplant 1996;10:51-4

[30] Sasal J, Naimark D, Klassen J, et al. Late renal transplant failure: an adverse prognostic factor at initiation of peritoneal dialysis. Perit Dial Int 2001;21:405-10

[31] Jassal SV, Lok CE, Walele A, Bargman JM. Continued transplant immunosuppression may prolong survival after return to peritoneal dialysis: results of a decision analysis. Am J Kidney Dis 2002;40:178-83: published online , doi:S0272-6386(02)00022-7 [pii];10.1053/ajkd.2002.33927 [doi]

[32] Sezer S, Karakan S, Ozdemir Acar FN, Haberal M. Dialysis as a bridge therapy to renal transplantation: comparison of graft outcomes according to mode of dialysis treatment. Transplant Proc 2011;43:485-7: published online , doi:S0041-1345(11)00028-5 [pii];10.1016/j.transproceed.2011.01.027 [doi]

[33] Perez FM, Rodriguez-Carmona A, Bouza P, et al. Delayed graft function after renal transplantation in patients undergoing peritoneal dialysis and hemodialysis. Adv Perit Dial 1996;12:101-4

[34] Van Biesen W, Vanholder R, Van Loo A, et al. Peritoneal dialysis favorably influences early graft function after renal transplantation compared to hemodialysis. Transplantation 2000;69:508-14

[35] Lobbedez T, Rognant N, Hurault dL, et al. Impact of automated peritoneal dialysis on initial graft function after renal transplantation. Adv Perit Dial 2005;21:90-3

[36] Freitas C, Fructuoso M, Martins LS, et al. Posttransplant outcomes of peritoneal dialysis versus hemodialysis patients. Transplant Proc 2011;43:113-6: published online , doi:S0041-1345(10)01910-X [pii];10.1016/j.transproceed.2010.12.008 [doi]

[37] Vanholder R, Heering P, Loo AV, et al. Reduced incidence of acute renal graft failure in patients treated with peritoneal dialysis compared with hemodialysis. Am J Kidney Dis 1999;33:934-40

[38] Bleyer AJ, Burkart JM, Russell GB, Adams PL. Dialysis modality and delayed graft function after cadaveric renal transplantation. J Am Soc Nephrol 1999;10:154-9

[39] Snyder JJ, Kasiske BL, Gilbertson DT, Collins AJ. A comparison of transplant outcomes in peritoneal and hemodialysis patients. Kidney Int 2002;62:1423-30

Kidney and Pancreas Transplantation: The History of Surgical Techniques and Immunosuppression

Jean-Paul Squifflet

Additional information is available at the end of the chapter

1. Introduction

Pancreas Transplantation aims at providing Beta cells replacement in diabetic patients, especially for type 1 diabetes recipients in whom Beta cells had been destroyed by an autoimmune process. The final achievement is to restore a normal physiological control of glucose metabolism in order to halt or reverse the secondary complications of diabetes i.e. retinopathy, neuropathy, nephropathy, micro – and macro - angiopathy [1]. That can be achieved by a vascularised pancreas graft (referred as Pancreas Transplantation, PT) or by islet grafting (referred as Islet Transplantation, IT). The former PT includes transplanting 95% of unuseful cells, the exocrine part from one pancreas, while the last one IP, embolizing into the recipient liver, Islets of Langerhans after digestion and purification of several human pancreases. Three types of PT can be performed: the pancreas and a kidney are simultaneously transplanted with a single induction of immunosuppression (IS) therapy in hoping to correct both uremia and diabetes mellitus (SPK = Simultaneous Pancreas and Kidney Transplantation); the pancreas is transplanted after a successful kidney graft allowing two induction therapies along with the basic IS treatment (PAK = Pancreas After Kidney Transplantation) ; and finally the Pancreas can be transplanted alone in pre-uremic recipients with unawareness hypoglycaemic events or with rapidly evolving secondary complications of diabetes such as proliferative retinopathy, or advanced neuropathy (PTA = Pancreas Transplantation Alone) [1].

Moreover, in SPK, both organs the Pancreas and the Kidney are procured from the same deceased donor, either donor after brain death (DBD) or donor after cardiac death (DCD). In some US institutions, a segmental pancreas and the left kidney, are procured in a living donor [2], using a laparoscopic approach in the more recent year [3]. For PAK, in order to avoid an excessive IS load and two induction therapies, other institutions had proposed whenever possible to keep in stand-by the potential live kidney donor until a cadaver whole pancreatic compatible graft is available [1]. By contrast, the number of PTA remains limited in non uremic recipients with life-threatening complications of diabetes, in whom one might hope to avoid the hypoglycaemic events with a successful graft. That can also be achieved with IT. But except for rare cases, insulin independence with IT requires more than a single human pancreas and is limited over time [1]. Moreover, IT needs costly materials, chambers and rooms for preparation. That's why IT will not be included in the present report.

2. The history of surgical techniques in pancreas transplantation

The first pancreas transplantation performed by W. Kelly and R. Lillehei on December 17, 1966 at the University of Minnesota was a duct ligated segmental graft which was implanted in the left iliac fossa along with a kidney coming from the same cadaver donor in a 28 year old female uremic recipient with type 1 diabetic nephropathy [4]. It was the first ever SPK (Fig 1). The recipient was insulin-free for six days; later she needed exogenous insulin, the need being attributed to the high doses of steroids given to prevent rejection. However, she also developed graft pancreatitis, that was most likely related to duct ligation, and for which she received 950 Rads graft irradiation. On February 14, 1967, Kelly and Lillehei removed the pancreas and rejected kidney. The recipient died from pulmonary embolism 13 days after pancreas graft removal [4]. This first case exemplified many of the problems that were associated with TP over the following 2 decades: surgical complications, wound infections, and graft rejection.

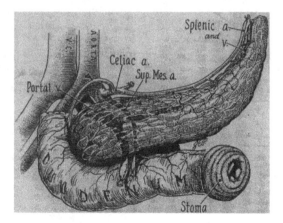

Figure 1. Drawing of the first segmental pancreas transplant (from Kelly et al.) [4].

Lillehei was the lead surgeon in the second pancreas transplant, also done with a kidney (Fig 2). He went on to do a total of 13 cases between the first case of Kelly and 1973, 9 with a kidney and 4 without [5, 6]. Significant changes in surgical techniques were made between the first and the second transplant pertaining to graft size (whole organ versus segmental) and duct management (cutaneous duodenostomy versus duct ligation). Lillehei transplanted the donor's whole pancreas and attached duodenum extraperitoneally to the 32-Year-old recipient's left iliac fossa (Fig 2). This transplant achieved a more prolonged state of graft function, but rejection treatment had to be instituted three and eight weeks post-transplant. Both rejection episodes affected the graft duodenum. The recipient was on insulin when she died four months post transplant from sepsis.

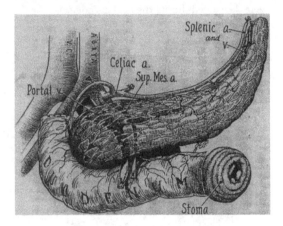

Figure 2. Drawing of the first whole pancreas transplant with cutaneous graft duodenostomy (from Lillelei et al.) [5]

After that series of 13 Pancreas Transplants, R. Lillehei concluded that most complications were associated with kidney graft rejection without pancreas rejection and recipient death [5, 6, 7].

After the first four pancreas transplants at the University of Minnesota, the next four transplants were performed in South America in 1968; [8, 9, 10]; three were performed in Brazil and one in Argentina at the Buenos Aires Hospital. Only one functioned sufficiently to induce insulin-independence and was subsequently lost to rejection at 4 months. [10].

In 1969, two other U.S. institutions performed one SPK transplant each: one at the University of Colorado (Fred Merkel and Thomas Starzl) and one at the University of California, Irvine Medical Center (John Connolly). [8, 11]. The first pancreas transplant in Europe, along with a kidney transplant, was performed in 1972 at Guys Hospital, in London, U.K. (Mick Bewick). [8].

By the 1970s, only 25 pancreas transplants had been performed at six institutions worldwide. Two-thirds of those early pancreas transplants were done along with a simultaneous kidney transplant. Exocrine secretions had been drained by duct ligation, cutaneous duodenostomy, or enteric drainage using a Roux-en-Y loop. Of these 25 grafts, only one, from Lillehei's original series, functioned for almost one year, and none for more than one year.

On November 24, 1971, Marvin Gliedman at Montefiore Hospital and Medical Center in New York performed the first pancreas transplant using urinary drainage via the native ureter [12]. Gliedman and associates performed a total of 11 ureteral pancreas transplants in the early 1970s (Fig 3) with one graft functioning for 22 months and another for 50 months – at that point the longest pancreas graft survival recorded. [13, 14]. However, ureteral drainage did not find widespread application because of tenuous leakage-prone duct-to-ureter anastomosis; leakage from the pancreas cut surface; and the potential need for ipsilateral native nephrectomy. The main conclusion drawn from that original and historical series was the probable evidence of a hierarchy in rejection, the pancreas being less antigenic than the kidney the latter being less antigenic than the duodenum [15]. Therefore, surgical techniques using a segmental pancreatic graft (body and tail) were developed during the next decade.

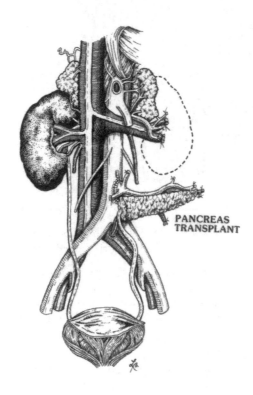

Figure 3. Ureteral pancreas transplant according to Gliedman et al [12] end-to-end distal ureter to pancreatic duct anastomosis.

2.1. The segmental pancreas transplantation reign (from mid 70's to mid's 80's)

In the mid 70's, the segmental pancreas while avoiding the duodenal segment was the most popular technique used for PT [6, 7]. Various procedures were proposed to drain the exocrine secretion: the duct could be left opened with the segmental graft placed intraperitoneally (Fig 4) [16] or blocked by an intraductal injection (Fig 5) of either Neoprene (J.M. Dubernard) [17] or Prolamine (W. Land) [18] or Polyisoprene (P. McMaster) [19] or Silicone (D.E.R. Sutherland) [20].

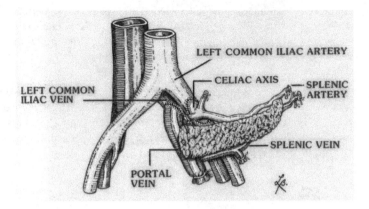

Figure 4. Technique for revascularization in the recipient of a segmental pancreas graft. The celiac axis (on a Carrel patch) and portal vein of the graft are anastomosed to the commun iliac vessels of the recipient through the meso-sigmoid [16].

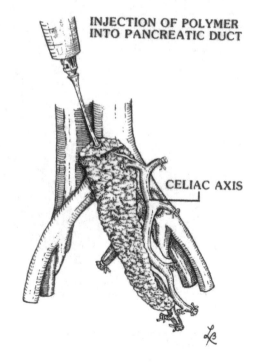

Figure 5. Injection of a synthetic polymer into the duct of a segmental pancreas graft following revascularization. Approximately 4-6 ml of the polymer is injected, followed by ligation of the duct [17-20].

Twelve intraperitoneal open-duct segmental pancreas transplants were performed at the University of Minnesota in a two-year period [16]; four were rejected within 4 months; 3 had to be removed because of peritonitis or ascites. The latter recipient lived insulin-independent for 18 years until in 1996 she died from a trauma, with a functioning graft, the longest duration of function at that time [21].

By contrast the duct occlusion technique became more popular despite numerous leaks, pancreatic fistulae, graft pancreatitis and vascular thrombosis. For managing these complications, Dubernard et al. [17, 7] proposed the omentoplasty in warping the duct-occluted segmental pancreas with the omentum, while Calne et al. [6, 7] was performing an A-V fistula at the distal end of the pancreas tail (Fig 6; panels A and B).

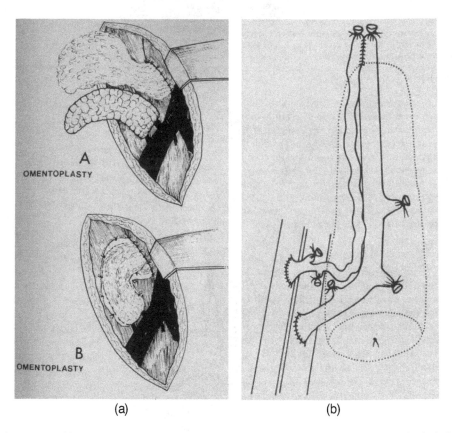

(a)   (b)

Figure 6. Panel (a): omentoplasty according to Dubernard et al.[7, 17]. Panel (b): AV fistula between the distal splenic artery and vein according to Calne et al. [6, 7].

During the late 70'S, three major events occurred that contributed to the development of PT.

Firstly, in 1979, the clinical use of Cyclosporine A (CsA) by R. Calne et al. [22] as the single immunosuppressant in 36 recipients of cadaveric organs. CsA remained the basic immunosuppressive (IS) drug up to the early 90'S.

Secondly, in 1980, the organization by J.M. Dubernard in Lyon, France, of the first pancreas transplantation meeting, launching the International Pancreas (and Islet) Transplant Registry (IPTR) which was handled by D.E.R. Sutherland at the University of Minnesota [23].

Thirdly and finally, in 1981, the first of a series of 5 workshops – called the Spitzingsee Meeting – organized by W. Land in Kühtai, Austria [24]. The characteristics of these workshops consisted in gathering the world pioneers in PT and allowing them to discuss on not only the successes but also the failures, finding ways to prevent them or improve the results [25]. These meetings were also the basis of creating the International Pancreas and Islet Association (IPITA) and later on, in Europ, the European Study Group in Simultaneous Pancreas and Kidney Transplantation (EuroSPK) [25]. More recently, was created the EPITA, the European Pancreas and Islet Transplantation Association [25].

During one of these workshops, H. Sollinger [26] had the idea to renew an old technique and divert the exocrine secretion of the pancreas into the bladder (Fig 7), while G. Tyden [27] and C. Groth [28] were proposing the enteric drainage (Fig 8). Slowly, both groups moved from the segmental graft [28] to the whole pancreas graft along with a duodenal segment (Fig 9) [26, 27]. This announced the end of the segmental transplantation reign. In the mean time, on November 10, 1982, the first pancreas transplantation was performed in Belgium by J.P. Squifflet and G.P.J. Alexandre [7]. The recipient was a 29 year old female with a 26 year history of type 1 diabetes. She was on peritoneal dialysis since one year and switched to hemodialysis a month before. She received a simultaneous pancreas and kidney transplants from a 22 year old female cadaver donor who died in a car accident from a head trauma. The recipient did not share any HLA antigen with the donor. She received a segmental pancreas graft, anastomosed on a Roux-en-Y loop (Fig 10), according to the technique described by Groth et al. (Fig 8) [23]. The immunosuppressive therapy consisted in a short course of antilymphocytic globulins induction along with cyclosporine A and steroids. She was one of the first few patients who received cyclosporine A in Belgium, at a dose a 14 mgr/kg/day. Following an episode of delayed graft function of the kidney, she fully recovered and was insulin free for a period of 2 years. Than insulin resistance was noticed along with an increase of 15 kg in body weight. Despite Cyclosporin and steroids dose reduction and the introduction of azathioprine, insulin therapy was resumed. She eventually went back on hemodialysis 8 years later and died in June 1992 while waiting for a second kidney transplant. The choice of the surgical technique and IS was based on animal experiments [29–32] but also on the fact that segmental pancreas transplantation was more popular during that period.

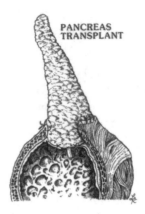

Figure 7. Exocrine secretion of segmental grafts drained directly into the bladder, as first described by Sollinger et al. [26].

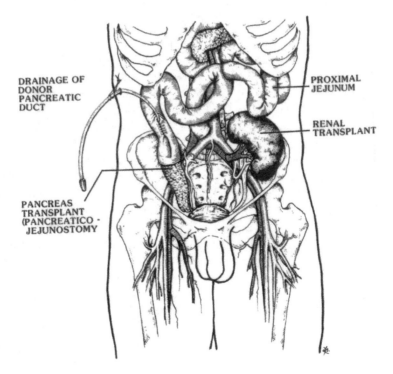

Figure 8. Enteric drainage of a segmental pancreas graft to a Roux-en-Y limb of recipient jejunum. The temporary external drainage of the pancreatic duct secretions to the catheter brought to the Roux-en-Y loop and the abdominal wall is illustrated [28].

2.2. The whole pancreas transplantation reign (from mid 80's)

Thus, in the mid 80's, whole pancreas transplantation with a duodenal segment became the gold standard surgical procedure.

In 1987, Nghiem and Corry at the University of Iowa described the technique of bladder drainage via a graft-to-recipient duodeno-cystostomy for whole pancreaticoduodenal grafts (Fig 9) [33]. Most U.S. and European centers quickly adopted bladder drainage via the graft duodenum. For SPK transplants, the dominant reason to use bladder-drainage was to reduce the risk of anastamotic leaks, since rejection could be monitored by serum creatinine. For solitary pancreas transplants, bladder-drainage had the advantage of urine amylase monitoring for rejection.

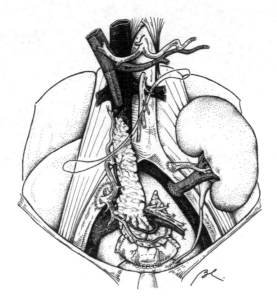

Figure 9. Pancreaticoduodenal transplantation with bladder drainage. A side-to-side anastomosis of the duodenal segment is made to the dome of the bladder [33].

In the mid 80's, Starzl [34] and associates reintroduced in U.S.the technique of enteric-drained whole-organ pancreaticoduodenal transplants, as originally described by Lillehei while the Stockholm group continued to do enteric drainage by direct duodeno-enterostomy [35]. Nearly everyone was convinced that whole pancreaticoduodenal transplants were preferable for PT from cadaver donors, and after en – bloc liver and pancreas procurement (Fig 11), transplant surgeons designed methods for reconstructing the vasculature to both organs (Fig 12) [36 - 39].

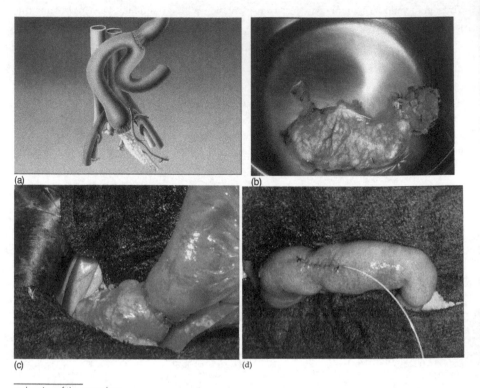

a: drawing of the procedure.
b: the segmental pancreas graft.
c: the end-to-end pancreas graft anastomosis to the Roux-en-Y loop.
d: the anastomosis suture was protected by a catheter inserted into the pancreas duct.

Figure 10. Segmental pancreatic transplant in the first Belgian recipient with enteric diversion of the exocrine secretion, in a Roux-en-Y loop.

From the mid-80s to the mid-90s, bladder drainage became the most common technique worldwide (Fig 9). However, because of chronic complications of bladder drainage (urinary tract infections, cystitis, urethritis (Fig 13), reflux pancreatitis, hematuria, metabolic acidosis and dehydration from fluid and bicarbonate losses), leading to conversion to enteric drainage in approximately a quarter of the recipients, in the mid-1990s, surgeons began to shifted to primary enteric drainage (Fig 14), not only for SPK transplants, but at some institutions also for solitary pancreas transplants [40].

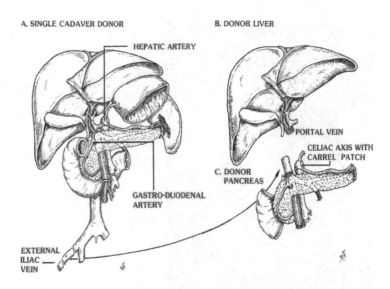

Figure 11. Maneuvers for en-bloc removal of a whole pancreas and a liver from a cadaver donor with normal vascular anatomy. The gastroduodenal artery must be divided so that the common and proper hepatic arteries can remain in continuity and be retained with the liver. The portal vein is divided just superior to the entrance of the splenic vein. Then, the pancreatic portion is lengthened by an iliac vein graft. The celiac and superior mesenteric arteries can remain with the pancreas with a Carrel aortic patch. [38]

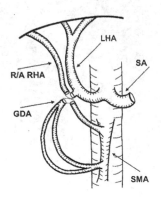

LHA = left hepatic artery.
GDA = gastroduodenal artery
SA = splenic artery
SMA = superior mesenteric artery.[39]

Figure 12. Whole-pancreas procurement and reconstruction of its arterial supply in a donor with a replaced / accessory right hepatic artery (R / A RHA).

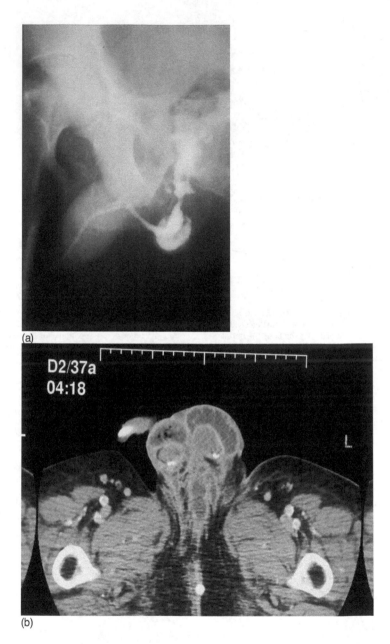

(a)

D2/37a
04:18

(b)

Figure 13. Chemical urethritis in a pancreas recipient with bladder drainage of the exocrine secretion (Panel (a)). CT scan: same recipient (Panel (b)).

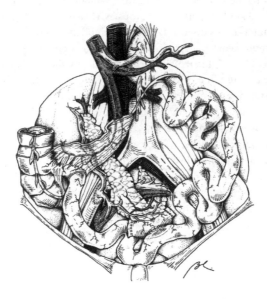

Figure 14. Pancreaticoduodenal transplantation with enteric drainage. A side-to-side anastomosis of the duodenal segment is made to the distal ileon, or the proximal jejeunum. It can also be performed on a Roux-en-Y loop [35].

2.3. The modern era of surgical techniques

Either enteric or bladder drainage is now done for virtually all pancreas transplants using a whole pancreas graft with a duodenal segment. The other techniques are virtually never used unless for salvage of a technical situation (e.g., duct injection might be used to manage a leak). With regard to the venous drainage of pancreas grafts, portal would be the most physiological but the systemic venous system was only accessed during the first two decades. Later on, the use of portal drainage at the junction of the recipient's superior mesenteric and splenic vein was favored in recipients of enteric drained whole-organ pancreaticoduodenal transplants (Fig 15). Surgeons reported on its metabolic and possible immunologic advantage, features also noted at the University of Maryland, where a large program existed of conversion to almost exclusive portal drainage [41]. By the end of the 1990's, almost 20 % of pancreas transplants in U.S. and in Europe were being done with portal drainage but the proportion did not increase nearly as much as the proportion of pancreas grafts that were enteric drained, reaching over 80 % for solitary in U.S. and over 90 % for SPK transplants in Europe (Fig 16). Early diagnosis of pancreas rejection had been difficult from the beginning, in particular for solitary pancreas transplants where serum creatinine could not be used as a surrogate marker like in SPK. That's why there is still room for improvement in surgical techniques. In order to have easy access to the graft for performing biopsies, De Roover et al. [42] proposed recently a technical modification and a side-to-side duodeno-duodenal (D-D) anastomosis while using a whole pancreaticoduodenal transplant with the venous effluent drained into the portal system of the recipient (Fig 17, 18). It offers serial sampling of the duodenal transplant mucosa by simple fibroscopies, a useful tool for monitoring rejection (Fig 18, Panel B). The duodenal anastomosis can be hand-made or performed using a stapler device. But the major drawback of both techniques could be the management of duodenal leaks on graft thrombosis. Our experience in 11 pancreas recipients at the University of Liege, CHU Sart Tilman is summarized in table 1. Peri-pancreatic collections, with or without pancreatitis were managed by surgical exploration and drainage. So far, only one graft thrombosis (PTA) needed prompt removal but was followed by a duodenal leak with cutaneous fistula which required weeks before healing (table 1). Therefore, prospective studies will be useful to specify the place of the D-D and each particular surgical suturing technique.

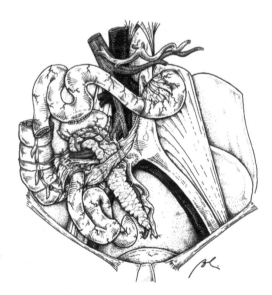

Figure 15. Pancreaticoduodenal transplantation with enteric drainage and portal drainage at the junction of the recipient's superior mesenteric and splenic veins [41].

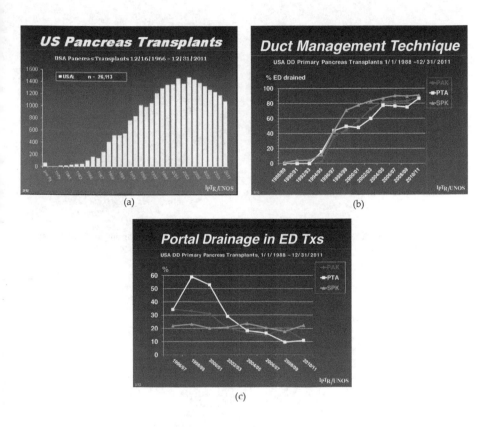

(a)

(b)

(c)

*By courtesy from A.E. Gruessner
Department of Surgery,
University of Arizona, Tucson, USA.

Figure 16. International Pancreas Transplant Registry * Panel (a): US Pancreas Transplants per year, between 12/16/1966 and 12/31/2011. Panel (b): Duct management techniques (urinary versus enteric drainage) in US primary pancreas transplants, between 1/1/1988 and 12/31/2011. Panel (c): Portal Drainage in enteric drained (ED) transplants. US primary pancreas transplants, between 1/1/1988 and 12/31/2011.

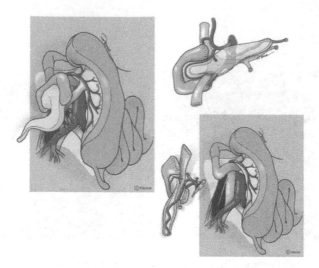

Figure 17. Pancreaticoduodenal transplantation with portal drainage and side-to-side recipient duodenal drainage of the exocrine secretion [23]: schematic representation and positioning.

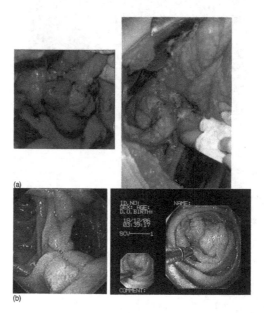

Figure 18. Pancreaticoduodenal transplantation with portal drainage and side-to-side recipient duodenal drainage of the exocrine secretion [23]: Panel (a): per operative view Panel (b): endoscopic view of the duodenum

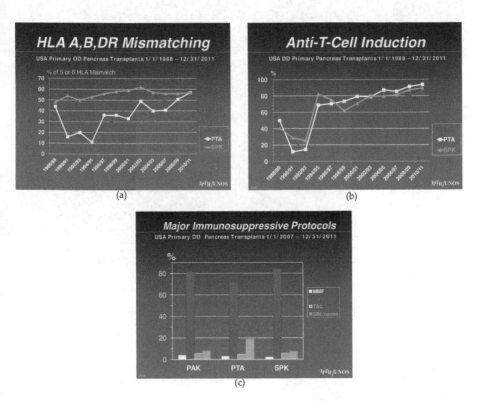

(a)

(b)

(c)

*By courtesy from A.E. Gruessner
Department of Surgery,
University of Arizona, Tucson, USA.

Figure 19. International Pancreas Transplant Registry* Panel (a): Purcentage of 5 or 6 HLA A, B, Dr Mismatching in US primary pancreas transplants between 1/1/1988 and 12/31/2011. Panel (b): Anti-T-Cell induction in US primary pancreas transplants between 1/1/1988 and 12/31/2011. Panel (c): Major immunosuppressive protocols in US primary pancreas transplants between 1/1/2007 and 12/31/2011

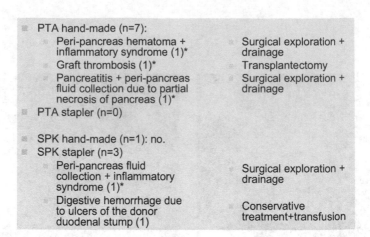

Table 1. Complications and outcome in 11 recipients of whole pancreas grafts with duodeno-duodenostomy, at the University of Liege, CHU Sart Tilman. The D-D anastomosis was hand-made (n=7) or using a stapler device (n=4)

3. The history of immunosuppression in pancreas transplantation

Advances in immunosuppressive protocols and the introduction of new immunosuppressants have had a major impact on and improved outcome after PT. As already mentioned, in 1979, Calne and associates first reported the successful use of cyclosporine in two pancreas recipients [22]. Due to the large dose of CsA used as a single agent and its nephrotoxicity, Starzl et al. proposed to combined reduced doses of CsA with steroids [43]. Further decreased in CsA dosages by using the synergistic effect of combining CsA to Aza was proposed by Squifflet et al. based on animals experiments [29, 44]. Triple drugs combining CsA, Aza and Steroids and later on quadruple drugs regimen with a short course induction of polyclonal Antibodies was the mainstay IS regimen during the next decade [21]. Starzl and his team first reported the use of Tacrolimus (Tac) in pancreas allograft recipients during the investigative period in 1989. [45] After approval, the first report on the use of Tac for pancreas transplantation was by D. Shaffer and associates, successfully reversing ongoing acute rejection in two SPK recipients. [46].

A major topic of the 4th Spitzingsee Workshop (January 30 – February 02, 1997; Kühtai, Austria) was the IS therapy in PT [25]. At that time, the newly introduced agent mycophenolate mofetil (MMF) was proved to be superior to azathioprine (Aza) for the prevention of acute rejection in kidney transplantation patients [47]. Data comparing Tac with the old (oil-based) formulation of CsA were also available in kidney transplantation, but there were some concerns about Tac having a diabetogenic effect [48], specially for pancreas. A preliminary study investigating the use of Tac in pancreatic transplantation, which was published by Gruessner et al., showed that pancreatic graft survival at 6 months post transplant was higher with Tac (79%) than in a historical group of SPK recipients treated with the oil-based formulation of CsA (65%; p = 0.04)

[49]. During the same era, the new micro-emulsion (Me) formulation of CsA (CsA – Me) had been introduced into clinical practice.

At that period, all European participants to the meeting were performing a limited number of SPK per centre. All realized that local studies would not aim solving the IS problems. Therefore W. Land took the opportunity to propose them the first large international prospective multicentre study in the field of PT, comparing Tac to the new CsA – Me, along with MMF, corticosteroids and a short course of induction therapy with Rabbit – antithymocyte globulines (R-ATG, Fresenius, Germany).

The rationale for induction therapy using anti-T-cell agents was triple: minimizing the risks of early rejection episodes, accelerating recovery of renal and pancreatic allograft function (protection against the ischemic reperfusion injury) and perhaps, inducing a tolerogenic effect to donor alloantigens. Before 1994, choices of maintenance IS agents were limited to a "one size fits all" approach with the combined use of Cyclosporin A (CsA), azathioprine (Aza) and corticosteroids. But, with that regimen, rejection rates were about 75 % to 80 %, with a rate of 25 % to 30 % of recurrence. Therefore, during the early 90's anti-T-cell induction was automatically added in all 3 categories of pancreas transplantation (Fig 19, Panel B). The choice of the anti-T-Cell agent was based more on its accessibility than on any rationale or scientific approach; the anti-T-Cell agents which were used are: MALG®, OKT3®, ATGAM®, R-ATG®, Simulect®, Zenapax®, Thymoglobulin®, Campath®. During the CsA era, single centre studies emphasized the benefit of Quadruple over Triple therapies [50, 51]. Other comparative studies underlined the best efficacy of ATG over OKT3® and MALG® [52 - 54]. During the modern era, during which most centres were using Tacrolimus (Tac), Mycophenolate Mofetil (MMF) and corticosteroids for maintenance therapy, Kaufman et al. designed several multicenter studies [55, 56] in which they confirmed the usefulness of induction therapy in PT. By contrast, the place of Campath®, still remains to be confirmed [57].

The results of the first Euro-SPK study were encouraging [58]. The 1-year incidence of biopsy-proven acute rejection of the kidney or pancreas was lower with Tac (27.2 %) than with CsA-Me (38.2 %; p = 0.09). Pancreatic graft survival at 1 year was significantly higher with Tac (91.3 %) than with CsA-Me (74.5 %; p = 0.0014). Kidney graft survival was similar in the two groups [58].

At 3 years, fewer patients receiving Tac (36.9 %) than CsA-Me (57.8 %) were discontinued from treatment (p = 0.003). The initial episodes of biopsy proven rejection were moderate or severe in just one out of 31 (3 %) Tac-treated patients compared with 11 of 39 (28 %) patients receiving CsA-Me (p = 0.009).

While 3-year patient and kidney survival rates were similar in the two treatment groups, pancreas survival was superior with Tac (89.2 vs 72.4 %; p = 0.002). Thrombosis resulted in pancreas graft loss in 10 patients receiving CsA-Me and in only 2 treated with Tac (p = 0.02). The overall incidence of adverse events was similar in both groups, but MMF intolerance was more frequent with Tac whereas hyperlipidaemia was more frequent with CsA-Me. Acute rejection was more common among CMV-infected patients (66 vs 41 % without infection; p = 0.001) and in those not receiving ganciclovir prophylaxis [48, 58].

7

There were no differences in 3-year kidney pancreas or patient survival between the 0-3 and 4-6 HLA antigen mismatch (MM) groups. Significantly more patients with 0-3 MM (66 %) were rejection-free at 3 years compared to those with 4-6 MM (41 %; p = 0.003). The relative risk of acute rejection was 2.6 times higher among patients with 4-6 MM than among those with 0-3 MM [48].

In summary the Euro-SPK study findings provided evidence to support the use of Tac in patients undergoing SPK transplantation.

A second SPK study addressed the issue of the choice of the antiproliferative agent which could be associated to Tac, either MMF or rapamycine (Rapa). Preliminary one and three year results demonstrated more frequent study withdrawal in the Rapa group, due to toxicity [59].

More than 60 % of those patients were rejection free at 1 year. Adequate kidney and pancreas functions were also achieved in both groups while the serum creatinine level was significantly lower in the Rapa group from month 2, the price to pay being hyperlipidemia, delayed wound healing, lymphocoele or hernia.

Corticosteroid withdrawal was possible in both studies in 70 % and 50 % of recipients respectively. Therefore, it can be concluded that steroid withdrawal is feasible in SPK trans-plantation but not in all patients; further studies must be designed to address that issue completely.

4. Conclusion

The current gold standard IS therapy for all three categories of pancreas transplantation includes induction with polyclonal antibodies and for the maintenance therapy, association of Tac with either MMF or Rapa, the last drug being less popular at least during the first postoperative period due to its possible side-effects (Fig 19).

Based on that potent IS therapy, functional results and patient survival rates of PT are coming closer to those currently achieved in kidney transplantation (Fig 20).

SPK transplantation remains the best therapeutic approach for type 1 diabetic recipients with (pre) end-stage renal failure (creatinine clearance < 50ml/min), up to 55 years of age, without any cardiovascular risk. They have three options: either waiting for the 2 grafts coming from the same -cadaver or live- donor, or one graft –usually the kidney – coming from a live donor who is in stand-by while waiting for the pancreas from a cadaver donor.

PAK can be offered to diabetic recipients who had the opportunity of having a live donor for kidney transplantation.

For other type 1 diabetic recipients, with (pre) end-stage renal failure, more than 55 years of age, with cardiovascular risk factors, they have 2 options: either receiving a kidney transplant alone (and eventually waiting for islet cells) or waiting for a simultaneous islet and kidney transplantation from the same cadaveric donor.

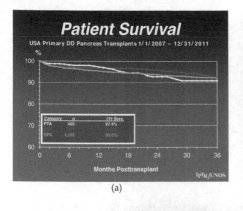
(a)

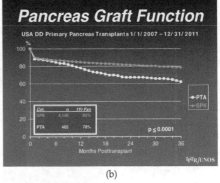
(b)

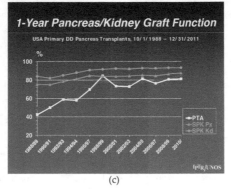
(c)

*By courtesy from A.E. Gruessner
Department of Surgery,
University of Arizona, Tucson, USA.

Figure 20. International Pancreas Transplant Registry* Panel (a): Patient survival in US primary pancreas transplants between 1/1/2007 and 12/31/2011. Panel (b): Pancreas graft function in all 3 categories (SPK, PAK, PTA). Panel (c): One year pancreas and kidney graft function in US primary pancreas transplants, between 10/1/1988 and 12/31/2011.

PTA should be considered for selected type 1 diabetic candidate without nephropathy, with hypoglycemia unawareness syndrom, with proliferative retinopathy. These candidates could be also candidates for islet transplantation, knowing the fact that they will be submitted to the same IS therapy and its long term deleterious side-effects in both options, they might also know that, with islet insulin independence is not always achieved.

Acknowledgements

- Drawings: to Benoit Lengele (BL) and Pierre Bonnet (PB).
- IPTR data : to A.E. Gruessner, and R.W.G. Gruessner, Departement of Surgery, University of Arizona, Tucson, USA.
- EuroSPK data : to all Members of the EuroSPK study group.

Author details

Jean-Paul Squifflet

Department of Abdominal Surgery and Transplantation, University of Liege, Belgium

References

[1] Pancreas transplantation White SA., Shaw J.A. and Sutherland D.E.R. Lancet (2009). , 373, 1808-17.

[2] Gruessner, R. W. G, Kendall, D. M, Drangstveit, M. B, Gruessner, A. C, & Sutherland, D. E. R. Simultaneous pancreas kidney transplantation from live donors Ann Surg (1997). , 226, 471-482.

[3] Gruessner, R. W. G, Kandaswamy, R, & Denny, R. Laparoscopic simultaneous nephrectomy and distal pancreatectomy from a live donor. J Am Cell Surg (2001). , 193, 333-337.

[4] Kelly, W. D, Lillehei, R. C, Merkel, F. K, & Idezuki, Y. And Goetz F.C. Allotransplantation of the pancreas and duodenum along with the kidney in diabetic nephrology. Surgery, (1967).

[5] Lillehei, R. C, Simmons, R. L, Najarian, J. S, Weil, R, Uchida, H, Ruiz, J. O, Kjellstrand, C. M, & Goetz, F. C. Pancreatico-duodenal allotransplantation : experimental and clinical experience. Ann Surg (1970). , 172, 405-436.

[6] Sutherland, D. E. R, & Gruessner, R. W. G. History of Pancreas Transplantation. in:Transplantation of the Pancreas Gruessner R.W.G. and Sutherland D.E.R. (eds), (2004). Springer- Verlag New York, Inc. , 39-68.

[7] Squifflet, J. P, Gruessner, R. W. G, & Sutherland, D. E. R. The history of Pancreas Transplantation: Past, Present and Future. Acta Chir Belg. (2008).

[8] Sutherland DERPancreas and islet transplantation. II. Clinical trials. Diabetologia (1981). , 20, 435-450.

[9] Sutherland DERPancreas and islet transplantation. II. Clinical trials. Diabetologia (1981)., 20, 435-450.

[10] Bortagaray, M. C, Zelasco, J. F, Bava, A, et al. Homotransplante parcial del pancreas en el diabetico. Pren Med Argent (1970).

[11] Connolly, J. E, Martin, R. C, Steinberg, J, et al. Clinical experience with pancreatico-duodenal transplantation. Arch Surg (1973)., 106, 489-493.

[12] Gliedman, M. L, Gold, M, Whittaker, J, Rifkin, H, Soberman, R, Freed, S, Tellis, V, & Veith, F. J. Clinical segmental pancreatic transplantation with ureter-pancreatic duct anastomosis for exocrine drainage. Surgery (1973)., 74, 171-180.

[13] Gliedman, M. L, Tellis, V. A, & Soberman, R. Long-term effects of pancreatic transplant function in patients with advanced juvenile onset diabetes. DiabetesCare (1978)., 1, 1-9.

[14] Tellis, V. A, Veith, F. J, & Gliedman, M. L. Ten-year experience with human pancreatic transplantation. Transplant Proc (1980). suppl 2):78-80.

[15] Lillehei, R. C, Ruiz, J. O, Aquino, C, & Goetz, F. C. Transplantation of the pancreas. Acta Endocrin (1976). suppl 205):303-320.

[16] Sutherland, D. E. R, Goetz, F. C, & Najarian, J. S. Intraperitoneal transplantation of immediately vascularized segmental grafts without duct ligation. A clinical Trial. Transplantation (1979)., 28, 485-491.

[17] Dubernard, J. M, Traeger, J, Neyra, P, Touraine, J. L, Traudiant, D, & Blanc-brunat, N. A new method of preparation of segmental pancreatic grafts for transplantation: Trials in dogs and in man. Surgery (1978)., 84, 633-640.

[18] Land, W, Gebhardt, C, Gall, F. P, Weitz, H, Gokel, M. J, & Stolte, M. Pancreatic duct obstruction with prolamine solution. Transplant Proc (1980). suppl 2): 72-75.

[19] Mcmaster, P, Calne, R. Y, Gibby, O. M, & Evans, D. B. Pancreatic transplantation. Transplant Proc (1980). suppl 2): 58-61.

[20] Sutherland, D. E. R, Goetz, F. C, Rynasiewicz, J. J, Baumgartner, D, White, D. C, El-ick, B. A, & Najarian, J. S. Segmental pancreas transplantation from living related and cadaver donors. Surgery (1981)., 90, 159-169.

[21] Sutherland, D. E. Gruessner RWG, Dunn DC, Matas AJ, Humar A, Kandaswamy R, Mauer SM, Kennedy WR, Goetz FC, Robertson RP, Gruessner AC, Najarian JS. Lessons learned from more than 1000 pancreas transplants at a single institution. Ann Surg (2000)., 233, 463-501.

[22] Calne, R. Y, Rolles, K, White, D. J. G, et al. Cyclosporine A initially as the only immunosuppressant in 36 recipients of cadaveric organs : 32 kidneys, 2 pancreas and 2 livers. Lancet (1979)., 2, 1033-1036.

[23] Sutherland, D. E. R. International Human Pancreas and Islet Transplant Registry. Transplant Proc (1980). suppl 2): 229-236.

[24] Land, W, & Landgraf, R. Segmental pancreatic transplantation international workshop Horm Metal Res (1983). , 13, 1-104.

[25] The History of the EuroSPK-Study Group, Squifflet J.P., Malaise J., Van Ophem D., Marcelis V. and Land W.G. Acta Chir Belg, (2008).

[26] Sollinger, H. W, Kamps, D, Cook, K, et al. Segmental pancreatic allotransplantation with pancreatico-cystostomy and high-dose cyclosporine and low-dose prednisone. Transplant Proc (1983). , 15, 2997-99.

[27] Tyden, G, Tibell, A, Sandberg, J, Brattstrom, C, & Groth, C. G. Improved results with a simplified technique for pancreaticoduodenal transplantation with enteric exocrine drainage. Clin Transplant (1996). , 10, 306-309.

[28] Groth, C. G, Collste, H, Lundgren, G, Wilczek, H, Klintmalm, G, Ringden, O, Gunnarsson, R, & Ostman, J. Successful outcome of segmental human pancreatic transplantation with enteric exocrine diversion after modifications in technique.Lancet (1982). , 2, 522-524.

[29] Squifflet, J. P, Sutherland, D. E. R, Rynasiewicz, J. J, Field, M. J, Heil, J. E, & Najarian, J. S. Combined immunosuppressive therapy with cyclosporine A and azathioprine. Transplantation (1982). , 34, 315-318.

[30] Squifflet, J. P, Sutherland, D. E. R, Morrow, C. E, Field, J, & Najarian, J. S. Comparison of rejection of intraportal islet versus immediately vascularized segmental Pancreatic allografts in rats in relation to beta cell mass engrafted. Transplant proc. (1983). , 15, 1344-1346.

[31] Squifflet, J. P, Sutherland, D. E. R, Florack, G, Morrow, C. E, & Najarian, J. S. Physiologic comparison of segmental pancreas and islet transplants in rats. Transplant Proc. (1985). , 17, 378-380.

[32] Squifflet, J. P, Sutherland, D. E. R, Florack, G, & Najarian, J. S. Pancreas Transplantation in the rat: long-term follow-up studies following different methods of management of exocrine drainage. Transplant Proc. (1986). , 18, 1143-1146.

[33] Nghiem, D. D, & Corry, R. J. Technique of simultaneous pancreaticoduodenal transplantation with urinary drainage of pancreatic secretion. Amer J Surg (1987). , 153, 405-406.

[34] Starzl, T. E, Iwatsuki, S, & Shaw, B. W. Jr. , Greene DA, Van Thiel DH, Nalesnik MA, Nusbacher J, Diliz-Pere H, Hakala TR. Pancreaticoduodenal transplantation in humans. Surg Gynecol Obstet (1984). , 159, 265-272.

[35] Tyden, G, Tibell, A, Sandberg, J, Brattstrom, C, & Groth, C. G. Improved results with a simplified technique for pancreaticoduodenal transplantation with enteric exocrine drainage. Clin Transplant (1996). , 10, 306-309.

[36] Sutherland DER, Moudry KC, Najarian JS. Pancreas transplantation. In: Cerilli J, ed. Organ Transplantation and Replacement, Philadelphia: J.B. Lippincott; (1987). , 1987, 535-574.

[37] Delmonico, F. L, Jenkins, R. L, & Auchincloss, H. Jr., Etienne T.J., Russell P.S., Monaco A.B., Cosimi A.B. Procurement of a whole pancreas and liver from the same cadaveric donor. Surgery (1989). , 105, 718-723.

[38] Squifflet, J. P, De Hemptinne, B, Gianello, P, et al. A new technique for en-bloc liver and pancreas harvesting. Transplant Proc (1990). , 22, 2070-71.

[39] Malaise, J, Mourad, M, Van Ophem, D, & Squifflet, J. P. Procurement of Liver and Pancreas Allografts in Donors with Repaced / Accessory right Hepatic Arteries. Transplantation (2005). , 79, 988-991.

[40] Gruessner, A. C, & Sutherland, D. E. R. Pancreas transplant outcomes for United States (US) and non-US cases as reported to the United Network for Organ Sharing (UNOS) and the International Pancreas Transplant Registry (IPTR) as of June 2004. Clin Transplant (2005). , 19, 433-455.

[41] Philosophe, B, Farney, A. C, Schweitzer, E, Colonna, J, Jarrell, B. E, & Bartlett, S. The superiority of portal venous drainage over systemic venous drainage in pancreas transplantation : a retrospective study. Ann Surg (2000). , 234, 689-695.

[42] Deroover, A, Coimbra, C, Detry, O, Van Kemseke, C, Squifflet, J. P, Honore, P, & Meurisse, M. Pancreas graft drainage in recipient duodenum : preliminary experience. Transplantation (2007). , 84, 795-7.

[43] Starzl, T. E, Weil, R, Iwatsuki, S, et al. The use of Cyclosporin A and Prednisone in cadaver transplantation. Surg Gynecol Olstet 180; 151 : 17.

[44] Squifflet, J. P, Sutherland, D. E. R, Field, M. J, Rynasiewicz, J. J, Heil, J. E, & Najarian, J. S. Synergistic immunosuppressive effect of cyclosporine A and azathioprine. Transplant Proc (1983). , 15, 520-522.

[45] Starzl, T. E, Todo, S, Fung, J, Demetris, A. J, Venkatarammn, R, & Jain, A. FK506 for liver, kidney and pancreas transplantation. Lancet (1989). , 2, 1000-1004.

[46] Shaffer, D, Simpson, M. A, Conway, P, et al. Normal pancreas allograft function following simultaneous pancreas kidney transplantation after rescue therapy with tacrolimus (FK506). Transplantation (1995). , 59, 1063-1066.

[47] The Tricontinental Mycophenolate Mofetil Renal Transplantation Study GroupA blinded, randomized clinical trial of mycophenolate mofetil for the prevention of

acute rejection in cadaveric renal transplantation. Transplantation (1996). , 61, 1029-1037.

[48] Malaise, J, Van Ophem, D, & Squifflet, J. P. and the EuroSPK Study Group. Simultaneous Pancreas-Kidney Transplantation in the European Clinical setting : a comprehensive evaluation of long-term outcomes. Nephrol Dial Transplant (2005). Suppl 2) : iiii62., 1.

[49] Gruessner, R. W, Sutherland, D. E. R, Drangstveit, M. B, Troppman, C, & Gruessner, A. C. Use of FK 506 in pancreas transplantation. Transplant Int (1996). Suppl 1): 5251-5257.

[50] Wadstrom, J, Brekke, B, Wramner, L, Ekberg, H, & Tyden, G. Triple versus Quadruple induction immunosuppression in pancreas transplantation. Transplant Proc (1995). , 27, 1317-1318.

[51] Cantarovich, D, Karam, G, Giral- Classe, M, Hourmant, M, Dantal, J, & Blancho, G. Le Normand L. and Soulillou J.P. Randomized comparison of triple therapy and antithymocyte globulin induction treatment after simultaneous pancreas-kidney transplantation. Kidney Int (1998). , 54, 1351-1356.

[52] Lefrancois, N, et al. Prophylactic polyclonal versus monoclonal antibodies in kidney and pancreas transplantation. Transplant Proc (1990). , 22, 632-633.

[53] Fasola, C. G, Hricik, D. E, & Schulak, J. A. Combined pancreas-kidney transplants using quadruple immunosuppressive therapy : a comparison between antilymphoblast and antithymocyte globulins. Transplant Proc (1995). , 27, 3135-3136.

[54] Stratta, R. J, Taylor, R. J, Weide, L. G, Sindhi, R, Sudan, D, Castaldo, P, Cushing, K. A, Frisbie, K, & Radio, S. J. A prospective randomized trial of OKT3 vs ATGAM induction therapy in pancreas transplantation recipients. Transplant Proc (1996). , 28, 917-918.

[55] Kaufman, D. B, Burke, G, Bruce, D, Sutherland, D. E. R, Johnson, C, Gaber, A. O, Merion, R, Schweitzer, E, Marsh, C, Alfrey, E, Leone, J, Concepion, W, Stegall, M, Gores, P, Danovitch, G, Tolzman, D, Scotellaro, P, Salm, K, Keller, A, & Fitzsimmons, W. E. The role of antibody induction in simultaneous pancreas kidney transplant patients receiving tacrolimus + mycophenolate mofetil immunosuppression. Transplantation (2000). S 206.

[56] Kaufman, D. B, & Burke, G. W. III, Bruce D.S., Johnson C.P., Gaber A.O., Sutherland D.E.R., Merion R.M., Gruber S.A., Schweitzer E., Leone J.P., Marsh C.L., Alfrey E., Concepcion W., Stegall M.D., Schulak J.A., Gores P.F., Benedetti E., Smith C., Henning A.K., Kuehnel F., King S., Fitzsimmons W.E. A prospective, randomized, multicenter trial of antibody induction therapy in simultaneous pancreas-kidney transplantation. Am J Transplant. (2003). , 3, 855-864.

[57] Farney, A, Rogers, J, Ashcroft, E, Hartmann, E, Hart, L, Doares, W, Moore, P, Jarett, A, Sundberg, A, Adams, P, & Stratta, R. Alemtuzumab Versus Rabbit Antithymocyte

Globulin Induction in Kidney and Pancreas Transplantation : A prospective Randomized Study. Am J Transplant (2007). Suppl 2) : 233 (330).

[58] Bechstein, W. O, Malaise, J, Saudek, F, et al. Efficacy and safety of tacrolimus compared with cyclosporine microemulsion in primary simultaneous pancreas-kidney transplantation : 1- year results of a large multicentre trial. Transplantation (2004). , 77, 1221-1228.

[59] Pratschke, J, Malaise, J, Saudek, F, Margreiter, R, Arbogast, H, Fernandez-cruz, L, Pisarski, P, Viebahn, R, Peeters, P, Nakache, R, Berney, T, Vanrenterghem, Y, & Bechstein, W. and the EuroSPK Study Group. Sirolimus versus Mycophenolate Mofetil in Tacrolimus based primary simultaneous pancreas-kidney (SPK) Transplantation: 1 year results of a multicentre trial. Transplant Int (2007). Suppl 1): S 270.

Chapter 8

Pregnancy Post Transplant

Rubina Naqvi

Additional information is available at the end of the chapter

1. Introduction

Be a mother is natural desire in female belonging to any community world over. In most cultures, pregnant women have a special status in society and receive particularly gentle care. At the same time, they are subject to expectations that may exert great psychological pressure, such as having to produce a son and heir, and some societies increase female population to fulfill this demand. Rate of ovulation and thus fertility is decreased in female with end stage renal disease, even if pregnancy occurs in dialysis population, only about 23 % were successful till 1980s (European registry). Whereas, after successful renal transplantation not only fertility rate increases with reemergence of better ovulation, but rate of successful childbirth also increases to 70- 80 % (Naqvi 2006,Thopmson 2003).

In this chapter, we aim to review the course of pregnancy and its outcome in renal allograft recipients, in backdrop of different social and cultural values, which we face in this part of world.

2. Status of pregnancy related issues in country

The 2006-07 Pakistan Demographic and Health Survey (PDHS) was undertaken to address the monitoring and evaluation needs of maternal and child health and family planning programs. In 1992-96 marital fertility; reported as 7.6 children per married woman, with a decline of one child over the past decade, PDHS data 2006-2007 reports 6.6 children per married woman. Eight percent of ever-married women report that they had a miscarriage in the past five years; about 2 percent said they had an abortion, and 3 percent reported having a stillbirth. For the most recent five-year period preceding the survey, infant mortality is 78 deaths per 1,000 live births. In interpreting the mortality data, it is useful to keep in mind that sampling errors are quite large. For example, the 95 percent confidence intervals for the under-five mortality estimate of 94 per 1,000 are 86 and 103 per 1,000 indicating that, given the sample size of the 2006-07 PDHS, the true value may fall anywhere between 86 and 103 per 1,000 births. As observed in most studies, the mother's level of education is strongly linked to child survival. Higher levels of educational attainment are generally associated with lower mortality rates because education exposes mothers to information about better nutrition, use of contraceptives to space births, and knowledge about childhood illness and treatment. Similarly, childhood mortality rates decline as the wealth quintile increases. Only 34 percent of births in Pakistan take place in a health facility. Eleven percent is delivered in a public sector health facility and 23 percent in a private facility. Three out of five births (65 percent) take place at home. (Pakistan Demographic and Health Survey 2006-07, National Institute of Population Studies Islamabad, Pakistan. Macro International Inc. Calverton, Maryland USA, published June 2008)

The incidence of low birth weight (defined <2.5 Kg by WHO) in general population reported as high as 31% from South Asia (Badshah, 2008) and 33.9% reported from West Bengal, India. (Pahari 1997)

3. Status of renal transplant in country

The incidence of ESRD in Pakistan and neighboring country India would be expected to be higher since poor socioeconomic status predisposes the population to a number of infection-related glomerulonephritides and the incidence of nephrolithiasis is higher in both countries as they fall in a "stone belt."(Sakhuja, 2003) In addition 6.9 million people in country are affected by diabetes with the International Diabetes Federation estimating that this number will grow to 11.5 million by 2025. With low literacy rate and poor health facilities complications and end organ failure with diabetes and hypertension are more prevalent. If the incidence of ESRD is indeed 100 patients per million population per year, this would mean 18,000 patients for a population of 180 million in Pakistan. There are very few state run dialysis centers and most of them are small units with minimal care facilities, < 5 dialysis stations. The number of patients maintained on dialysis is likely to be < 50 patients per million population since few patients can afford this form of therapy. Sindh Institute of Urology and Transplantation (SIUT) is a semi government organization in country which cater largest population of patients suffering from any kind of kidney ailment. It is running largest hemodialysis and live related renal program not only in country but the region. This organization is unique in terms of providing free health care services to all, be it pre operative preparation, surgical procedure, life long follow up and immunosupression. (www.siut.org) Because of lack of state provided health facilities number of patients seen and treated at this hospital is beyond imagination and for same reason patients do comply during follow up and long term data from this institution is more reliable and representative.

Renal transplant started in country in 1979 from living related donors, initially the activity was as low as < 50 /year, which rose to about 2500 kidney transplants / year in 2007. Most of these were unrelated donor transplants done at private sector. In March 2010 Pakistan was fortunate to have been able to pass a viable and authentic transplant law and activity of unrelated donor transplant decreased. Deceased donor transplant yet has to take off in country, though few have been done from non heart beating donors, organs supplied by Euro-transplant foundation and five local deceased donors.

4. End Stage Renal Disease (ESRD) affecting fertility

Female with ESRD have hypothalamic-pituitary-gonadal dysfunction, associated with high follicle stimulating hormone, luteinizing hormone and prolactin levels. Ovulation is suppressed and mensturation is irregular. Additionally there is sexual dysfunction, suppressed desire and associated psychological factors resulting from chronic ailment. Women on dialysis if conceive present with challenges of worsening of blood pressure controls and anemia, and higher incidences or pre-eclampsia. In 1980, the European Dialysis and Transplant Association reported that only 23% of 115 pregnancies in dialysis ended with surviving infants (European Registry). In 1998, Bagon et al. described a national survey showing a successful outcome in approximately half of the pregnancies in dialysis patients. There are few case series in the new millennium, mainly from single experienced centers, many of which report a successful outcome rate of >70% (Romao 1998, Barua 2008). Our own experience is limited with very poor outcome. (Unpublished)

5. Pregnancy post transplant

Reversal of normal endocrine function has been reported within 4-6 months after renal transplantation. (Ha 1991, Ghafari 2008, McKay 2008) Thus kidney transplant offers best hope for ESRF patients who keen to conceive. First pregnancy in renal transplant recipient was reported by Murray in 1963, since then there are many published reports focusing on impact of pregnancy on renal graft outcome with a conclusion that pregnancy does not have an adverse effect on graft function provided recipient has stable graft function and no adverse event happens during pregnancy. (Table)

6. Optimal timing for pregnancy post transplant

Most transplant centers advise that women can conceive after 2 years of transplant provided graft function is stable i.e. serum creatinine is < 1.5 mg/dl and proteinuria <500 mg/day. At that time, risk of acute rejections generally low, immunosuppression has reduced to minimal, prophylactic anti bacterial and anti viral already completed and women are usually stable. All pregnancies should be considered as high risk and should be managed by multidisciplinary team.

Author	year	Duration	Country	No. of pregnancies reported	outcome
Cararach	1993	25 years	Spain	133	Abortions 10% Preterm 46% Full Term 53%
First	1995	23 years	USA	25	Abortions 3 Live births 22
Saber	1995	25 years	Brazil	25	Abortions 4 Preterm 14 Full term 7
Sturgiss	1996	23 years	UK	18 (compared with 18 non pregnant controls)	Long term graft survival compared in two groups.
Tan	2002	14 years	Singapore	42	Abortions 10 Still birth 1 Ectopic 2
Armenti	2004	14 years	USA NTPR	1125	Abortions 20% Still births 2.5% Ectopic 1% Premature births 53%
Kashanizadeh	2007	6 years	Iran	86	Abortions 24 Full term 62
Sibanda	2007	7 years	UK Transplant Pregnancy Registry	193	Abortions 32 IUDs 3 Ectopic 1 Live Births 149
Draihimh	2008	10 years	5 Middle East Countries	234	Abortions 19.3% Still births 7.3% Live births 74.4%
Naqvi	2010	24 years	Pakistan	68	Abortions 15 Preterm 8 Full term 45 (40 live, 5 IUD or FSB)

Table 1. Published results from world over

7. Risks for mother

Mothers who are renal transplant recipient have certain risks on graft function and survival. Many of renal transplant recipients have hypertension and some degree of renal dysfunction with GFR (Glomerular filtration rate) of not up to the mark, both are affected with pregnancy and blood pressure medications may require alterations and increment in dosages. Some may predispose to pre-eclampsia which is difficult to diagnose especially when few of these women already have some preexisting proteinuria and blood pressure frequently increases after 20th week of gestation. Poorly controlled hypertension can cause preterm delivery.

Women with preexisting graft dysfunction i.e. serum creatinine of > 1.5 mg/dl are at greater risk of developing irreversible worsening of graft function. (Davison 1976) Acute rejection can also occur as blood levels of immunosuppressant may alter with changing volume distribution during pregnancy, this phenomenon is more relevant with calcineurin inhibitors.(Donaldson 1996) However, available reports indicate that rejection rate in pregnant recipient not differ from non pregnant recipients. (Armenti 2004) In our experience of 68 pregnancies in renal transplant recipients, none experienced acute rejection during pregnancy. (Naqvi 2010)

Urinary tract infection rate also increases in pregnant renal transplant recipients, some have reported as high as 42%. (Oliveria 2007)

The transplant recipient is at increased risk for viral infections, therefore, maternal–fetal transmission of infectious agents needs to be considered as a potential risk not only to the mother but also to the fetus. Cytomegalovirus infection is particularly serious because it is associated with hearing/vision loss and mental retardation and can be transmitted from the mother to the fetus through a trans-placental route, as well as during delivery or in breast milk in case mother is feeding to infant. (del Mar Colon 2007, Ross 2006)

Other infections that may pose additional risks in the immunosuppressed mother include toxoplasmosis, primary herpes simplex infection, primary varicella infection, HIV infection, and infection with either hepatitis B or C virus (Gardella 2007, Shiono 2007)

As allograft recipients have increased risk for gestational diabetes, some have recommended that they should be screened every trimester with a 50-g oral glucose load. (del Mar Colon 2007)

8. Risks to fetus

Published reports from UK, USA and European registries persistently highlighted risk of low birth weight of fetus and pre term delivery in renal transplant recipients. (Sibanda 2007, Armenti 2004) Willis et al from Australia reported 44% with low birth weight. (Willis 2000) In our experience we found mean birth weight infants born to transplant recipients was 2.4± 0.57 Kg, with 7 newborns <1.8 Kg. (Naqvi 2010)

Exposure to immunosuppressants: Adrenal insufficiency and thymic hypoplasia have occasionally been described in the infants of transplant recipients, but these problems are unlikely if the dose of prednisone has been decreased to 15 mg (Penn I, 1980). Prednisolone traverses the placenta but 90 % of maternal dose is metabolized within the placenta and not reaching to fetus (Blanford 1977). In addition if pregnancy is occurring after 2 years of transplant, recipient already on very small dose of Prednisolone. Steroids can also aggravate hypertension in mother; mothers are more prone to infections if steroid dose is still high at time of conception. Premature rupture of membrane is another complication reported in relation of steroids. Therefore, it is recommended to get conceive when steroid dose is reduced to minimal. Reports from azathiaprine era through cyclosporine era have not identified specific malformations among infants born to transplant recipients (Armenti 2000). Radioactive labeling studies in humans have shown that 64–93% of Azathioprine administered to mothers appears in fetal blood as inactive metabolites (Sarikoski S, 1973). Cyclosporine metabolism appears to be increased during pregnancy and higher doses may be required to maintain plasma levels in the therapeutic range (Muirhead N, 1992). Data concerning the effect of tacrolimus on pregnancy is scarce. A report of 100 pregnant women (which included all organ transplant recipients), among 84 treated with tacrolimus, 68 progressed to a live birth, with 60% of deliveries being premature (Kainz A, 2000). Teratogenecity of mycophenolate mofetil is not yet confirmed, therefore it is recommended to switch over to azathiaprine in female who are planning to conceive. A study has reported low number of T and B cells at birth in infants born to mothers who were on immunosuppressants, but these were normalized after few months. (Di Paolo 2000) Most published studies related to subject have not described clear cut congenital malformations or autoimmune disorders to children born to transplant recipients, though sporadic case reports which could be related to exposure risk of disease in general population.

9. Breast feeding by transplant recipients

Sparse data is available on recommendations for breast feeding from immunosuppressant mothers. Study published on cyclosporine levels in breast milk reveals cyA levels in milk equivalent to mother's serum. (Moretti 2003) This leads to conclusion that females who are on cyclosporine should not fed their babies, whereas the fact that small amounts of azathiaprine and Prednisolone are excreted in milk (Coulam 1982) can provide an opportunity to consider feeding those babies whose mothers are on these two agents only. French et al. reported the first case of measurement of tacrolimus levels in human milk; suggest that maternal therapy with tacrolimus may be compatible with breast-feeding. (French 2003). Level of Tacrolimus was calculated in breast milk in this case but this was single case report. Data on other drugs is still lacking.

Recommendations

1.   preconception counseling is a must

2.   good general health for about 2 years after transplant

3. stature compatible with good obstetric outcome

4. no or minimal proteinuria

5. no hypertension or well controlled blood pressure on one agent

6. consider revising anti-hypertensive regimen when pregnant

7. no evidence of recent graft rejection

8. stable graft function with serum creatinine less than 1.5 mg/dl

9. drug therapy at maintenance levels

10. switch immunosuppressants to milder, e.g. MMF should be converted to AZA, Tacrolimus to CyA and Prednisolone in minimal doses

11. once pregnant, transplant recipient should be seen by multidisciplinary team with a frequency of 4 weeks during first trimester and 2 weeks later on.

Author details

Rubina Naqvi*

Nephrology Sindh Institute of Urology and Transplantation (SIUT), Karachi, Pakistan

References

[1] Armenti, V. T, Radomski, J. S, Moritz, M. J, Gaughan, W. J, Hecker, W. P, Lavelanet, A, & Mcgrory, C. H. Coscia LA: Report from the National Transplantation Pregnancy Registry (NTPR): Outcomes of pregnancy after transplantation. Clin.Trans, (2004). , 2004, 103-114.

[2] Bagon, J. A, Vernaeve, H, De Muylder, X, Lafontaine, J. J, Martens, J, & Van Roost, G. Pregnancy and dialysis. Am J Kidney Dis (1998). PubMed: 9590184], 31, 756-765.

[3] Barua, M, Hladunewich, M, Keunen, J, Pierratos, A, Mcfarlane, P, Sood, M, & Chan, C. T. Successful pregnancies on nocturnal home hemodialysis. Clin J Am Soc Nephrol (2008). PMCID: PMC2390936] [PubMed: 18308997], 3, 392-396.

[4] Badshah, S, Mason, L, Mckelvie, K, & Payne, R. Lisboa PJG; Risk factors for low birth weight in public hospitals at Peshawar, NWFP-Pakistan. BMC Public Health. (2008).

[5] Blanford, A. T, & Murphy, B. E. In vitro metabolism of prednisone, dexamethasone, and cortisol by the human placenta. Am J Obstet Gynecol (1977). , 127, 264-7.

[6] Cararach, V, Carmona, F, Monleon, F. J, & Andreu, J. Pregnancy after renal transplantation: 25 years experience in Spain. Br J Obstet Gynaecol. (1993).

[7] Coulam, C. B, Moyer, T. P, Jiang, N. S, & Zincke, H. Breast-feeding after renal transplantation. Transplant Proc (1982). , 14, 605-9.

[8] Donaldson, S, Novotny, D, Paradowski, L, & Aris, R. Acute and chronic lung allograft rejection during pregnancy. Chest (1996). , 110, 293-6.

[9] Di Paolo SSchena A, Morrone LF, Manfredi G, Stallone G, Derosa C, Procino A, Schena FP. Immunologic evaluation during the first year of life of infants born to cyclosporine-treated female kidney transplant recipients: analysis of lymphocyte subpopulations and immunoglobulin serum levels. Transplantation (2000). , 69, 2049-54.

[10] Davison, J. M, & Lind, T. Uldall PR: Planned pregnancy in a renal transplant recipient. Br J Obstet Gynaecol,(1976).

[11] Draihimh, H. A, Ghamdi, G, Moussa, D, Shaheen, F, Mohsen, N, Sharma, U, Stephan, A, Alfie, A, Alamin, M, Haberal, M, Saeed, B, & Kechrid, M. Al-Sayyari A; Outcome of 234 pregnancies in 140 Renal Transplant Recipients from Five Middle Eastern Countries. Transplantation, (2008).

[12] del Mar Colon MHibbard JU: Obstetric considerations in the management of pregnancy in kidney transplant recipients. Adv Chronic Kidney Dis (2007).

[13] European Best Practice Guidelines IVPregnancy in renal transplant recipients. Nephrol Dial Transplant. (2002). suppl.4): 50-5.

[14] French, A. E, Soldin, S. J, Soldin, O. P, et al. Milk transfer and neonatal safety of tacrolimus. Ann. Pharmacotherapy. (2003). , 37(6), 815-8.

[15] First, M. R, Combs, C. A, & Weiskittel, P. Miodovnik M; Lack of Effect of Pregnancy on Renal Allograft Survival or Function. Transplantation. (1995).

[16] Ghafari, A. Sanadgol H; Pregnancy After Renal Transplantation: Ten-Year Single Center Experience. Trans Proc (2008).

[17] Gardella, C. Brown ZA: Managing varicella zoster infection in pregnancy. Cleve Clin J Med 74: 290-296, (2007).

[18] Kainz, A, Harabacz, I, Cowirick, I. S, & Gadgil, S. D. Haqiwara D; Review of the course and outcome of 100 pregnancies in 84 women treated with tacrolimus. Transplantation(2000). , 70, 1718-1721.

[19] Kashanizadeh, N, Nemati, E, Sharifi-bonab, M, Moghani-lankarani, M, Ghazizadeh, S, Einollahi, B, & Lessan-pezeshki, M. Khedmat H; Impact of Pregnancy on the Outcome of Kidney Transplantation. Trans Proceed. (2007).

[20] Moretti, M. E, Sgro, M, Johnson, D. W, Sauve, R. S, Woolgar, M. J, Taddio, A, Verjee, Z, Giesbrecht, E, Koren, G, & Ito, S. Cyclosporine excretion into breast milk. Transplantation (2003). , 75(12), 2144-6.

[21] Muirhead, N, Sabharwal, A. R, Reider, M. J, & Lazarovits, A. I. Hollomby DJ; The outcome of pregnancy following renal transplantation-the experience of a single center.Transplantation(1992). , 54, 429-432.

[22] Naqvi, R. Obstetrics in Renal Transplantation: A Series of Cases of Pregnancy Post Transplant Observed Over 24 Years. WebmedCentral TRANSPLANTATION (2010). WMC00950

[23] Naqvi, R, Noor, H, Ambareen, S, Khan, H, Haider, A, Jafri, N, Alam, A, Aziz, R, Manzoor, K, Aziz, T, Ahmed, E, Akhtar, F, & Naqvi, A. Rizvi A; Outcome of Pregnancy in Renal Allograft Recipients: SIUT Experience. Trans Proceed. (2006).

[24] Oliveira, L. S, Sass, N, Sato, J. L, & Ozaki, K. S. Medina Pestana JO; Pregnancy after renal transplantation: A five year single center experience. Clin Transplant (2007).

[25] Penn, I, Makowski, E. L, & Harris, P. Parenthood following renal transplantation. Kidney Int(1980). , 18, 221-223.

[26] Pahari, K, & Ghosh, A. Study of pregnancy outcome over a period of five years in a postgraduate institute of west Bengal. J Indian Med Assoc. (1997). Jun;, 95(6), 172-4.

[27] Ross, D. S, Dollard, S. C, Victor, M, & Sumartojo, E. Cannon MJ: The epidemiology and prevention of congenital cytomegalovirus infection and disease: Activities of the Centers for Disease Control and Prevention Workgroup. J Womens Health (Larchmt) (2006).

[28] Romão, J. E. Jr, Luders C, Kahhale S, Pascoal IJ, Abensur H, Sabbaga E, Zugaib M, Marcondes M.: Pregnancy in women on chronic dialysis. Nephron (1998). PubMed: 9580542], 78, 416-422.

[29] Successful pregnancies in women treated by dialysis and kidney transplantation: Report from the Registration Committee of the European Dialysis and Transplant AssociationBr J Obstet Gynaecol (1980). PubMed: 7000160], 87, 839-845.

[30] Sibanda, N, Briggs, J. D, Davison, J. M, & Johnson, R. J. Rudge CJ; Pregnancy After Organ Transplantation: A Report From the UK Transplant Pregnancy Registry. Transplantation. (2007).

[31] Sarikoski, S, & Seppala, M. Immunosuppression during pregnancy: transmission of azathioprine and its metabolites from the mother to the fetus. Am J Obstet Gynecol. (1973).

[32] Sakhuja, V, & Sud, K. End stage renal disease in India and Pakistan: burden of disease and management issues. Kidney Int. (2003). Suppl 83):SS118., 115.

[33] Shiono, Y, Mun, H. S, He, N, Nakazaki, Y, Fang, H, Furuya, M, & Aosai, F. Yano A: Maternal-fetal transmission of Toxoplasma gondii in interferon-gamma deficient pregnant mice. Parasitol Int 56: 141-148, (2007).

[34] Sturgiss, S. N. Davison JM; Effect of Pregnancy on the Long-Term Function of Renal Allograft: An Update. Am J Kid Dis. (1996).

[35] Saber LTSDuarte G, Costa JAC, Cologna AJ, Garcia TMP, Ferraz AS; Pregnancy and Kidney Transplantation: Experience in a Developing Country. Am J Kid Dis. (1995).

[36] Thompson, B. C, Kingdon, E. J, Tuck, S. M, & Fernando, O. N. Sweny P; Pregnancy in renal transplant recipients: the Royal Free Hospital experience. Q J Med. (2003).

[37] Tan, P. K, Tan, A. S, Tan, H. K, Vathsala, A, & Tay, S. K. Pregnancy after renal transplantation: experience in Singapore General Hospital. Ann Acad med Singapore, (2002).

[38] Willis, F. R, Findlay, C. A, Gorrie, M. J, Watson, M. A, Wilkinson, A. G, & Beattie, T. J. Children of renal transplant recipient mothers. J Paediatr Child Health. (2000). Jun;, 36(3), 230-5.

Chapter 9

Practical Pharmacogenetics and Single Nucleotide Polymorphisms (SNPs) in Renal Transplantation

María José Herrero, Virginia Bosó, Luis Rojas,
Sergio Bea, Jaime Sánchez Plumed, Julio Hernández,
Jose Luis Poveda and Salvador F. Aliño

Additional information is available at the end of the chapter

1. Introduction

Optimizing balance between therapeutic efficacy and the occurrence of adverse events is the main goal of individualized medicine. This takes even more importance in narrow therapeutic index drugs such as immunosuppressants. These drugs are highly effective in preventing acute graft rejection but tacrolimus, cyclosporine and mycophenolic acid show highly variable pharmacokinetics and pharmacodynamics. Still nowadays the fragile equilibrium between the risks and benefits of immunosuppression makes the management of immunosuppressive pharmacotherapy a challenge.

Therapeutic drug monitoring (TDM) is an essential and indispensable instrument for calcineurin inhibitors dosing, reducing the pharmacokinetic component of variability by controlling drug blood concentrations. But TDM is only possible once the drug is administered and steady state and patient's compliance are achieved, so complementary strategies are needed. Moreover, despite correct TDM, it may take several days or even weeks to reach target blood concentrations. For many patients this time periods are not appropriate in order to achieve sufficiently high concentrations to prevent graft rejection or adverse reactions or, on the other hand, without exposing the patient to excessive toxicity. In this sense, Pharmacogenetics is an interesting approach, helpful to manage immunosuppressant drugs. Changes in expression or function of proteins and enzymes involved in drug transport, metabolism or mechanism of action will cause changes in drug's absorption, metabolism and distribution and, therefore, can lead to changes in the response and toxicity of the treatment. Characterization of these genetic variants, mainly Single Nucleotide Polymorphisms (SNPs), can help to establish effective doses and to minimize adverse effects. Many publications, including our own, have found statistically significant correlations between (SNPs) and tacrolimus and/or cyclosporine dose-corrected blood levels. There are also works correlating certain variants in SNPs with safety and efficacy of the treatment. Even some researchers, working groups and consortia recommend guidelines for initial dosing adjust regarding this SNPs.

Pharmacogenetic tests are becoming cheaper every day, so the cost of performing these assays is getting more assumable, especially when clinically relevant complications are demonstrated. The incorporation of pharmacogenetic studies to the real clinical practice will depend on the creation of well-designed sets of SNPs that, in a cost-effectiveness manner, could correlate clinical complications with genotypes, taking into consideration the whole and complicated treatment in polymedicated patients. Many results contribute to highlight the need of prospective controlled studies, with pharmacogenetic analysis prior to transplantation. This will probably be the critical point for the regulatory agencies to settle the most relevant polymorphisms as validated biomarkers to be widely used in the clinical transplantation setting.

For all this reasons, our aim in this chapter is to provide an easy explanation about what a polymorphism is and an updated view of the most relevant SNPs with evidence of their implication in safety and efficacy of immunosuppressive treatment in renal transplantation. The final goal is to give a summary from basic knowledge to concrete examples that help to improve the medical doctors' knowledge of the clinical impact of Pharmacogenetics in their daily practice.

2. Personalized medicine and pharmacogenetics

The term "Personalized Medicine" was not long ago some "scifi" concept, just expressing the best wishes of the scientific community with an aim of adjusting the pharmacotherapy as best as possible to each single patient. However, in the last years we have seen real advances in this area that have brought to the real clinical practice in most of the "first world" countries, a set of new analysis under the same principle: offering an individualized therapy to each different patient.

In order to understand this new approach in medicine and put it into practice, we necessarily have to take genetics in consideration, and particularly, we have to pay attention to the individual differences that make each patient respond in a different way to a given pharmacological treatment. Here, we arrive to the concepts of Pharmacogenetics and Pharmacogenomics, that can be heard in more and more places each day. They are, and for sure will be, components to be considered in the medical practice. We can define them in many ways, and traditionally they have been employed interchangeably although there are differences between them. They are different but complementary disciplines. The European Medicines Agency, EMA, takes their definitions from The International Conference on Harmonisation of Technical Requirements for Registration of Pharmaceuticals for Human Use (ICH), this is a project with regulatory authorities from Europe, Japan and USA, together with experts from pharmaceuticals that discusses technical and scientific aspects about the products registries. One of its aims is to reach a better harmonization in the interpretation and application of technical guides and requirements for the registries. ICH defines Pharmacogenomics as the study of variations in DNA and RNA characteristics regarding the response to drugs and it defines Pharmacogenetics as a subset inside pharmacogenomics, that studies the variations in the DNA sequence regarding the response to drugs [1-5].

There is another term that is also frequently found: biomarker, genetic or genomic biomarker, whose definition is "a measurable characteristic of DNA and/or RNA which is an indicator of a biological process that can be normal, pathogenic and/or a response to a therapeutic (or other kind) intervention. A genomic biomarker could be, for instance, the measuremente of a gene expression or of its regulation. It can consist in one or more DNA and/or RNA characteristics, as for instance, in DNA, its single nucleotide polymorphisms (SNPs); the variability in the repetition of short sequences; the haplotypes; DNA modifications as methilation; the deletions or insertions of a single nucleotide; the copy number variation; or the cytogenetic rearrangements as translocations, duplications, deletions or inversions. Regarding RNA, it could be a particular trait of its sequence; the levels of expression; the processing (as splicing and editing); or the levels of microRNAs. A deeper explanation of some of these terms will be done in the next paragraph.

The aim of pharmacogenomics is to identify the most important genetic elements in the instauration and/or evolution of a pathological process in order to create new strategies for drug evaluation and optimization of the drug development process. These are usually high throughput studies, regarding the simple number and statistical signification but also very exigent with the study subject: the final goal is finding correlation with the disease at a genomic level, not with one single nucleotide but with genes or groups of related genes instead. On the other side, pharmacogenetics studies the influence of genetic factors on the activity of a drug, making attention in concrete changes inside a gene that somehow has already been postulated as a candidate gene, by previous knowledge or by pharmacogenomic studies. Subject of pharmacogenetic studies are especially, the variants in genes related with transport and metabolism of drugs, with the aim that specific drugs can be given to specific groups of genetically defined (or "stratified") patients [6, 7].

To summarize, pharmacogenetics has to be considered as one of the mainstays of personalized medicine, which will let us correlate good or bad response to a drug in a specific population with genetic aspects. It will also let us know which drugs will offer greater therapeutic benefit or lower risk of adverse reactions development for a given population.

3. What are genetic polymorphisms?

We also must review some other basic concepts in genetics and, extensively, pharmacogenetics in order to understand the following information. The most relevant one is Polymorphism, which is defined as a mendelian monogenic character that appears in the population with the presence of more than one allele in the same genetic locus. Applying the term to pharmacogenetics, it makes reference to the different alleles or variants of a gene related to a drug interaction with the body. The frequency of the less common allele in the population must not be higher than 1%. The two main groups of genetic polymorphisms are Single Nucleotide Polymorphisms (SNPs) and Lenght Polymorphisms (repetitions of nucleotide groups). The first group represents 90% of genetic variability in our genome, and each nucleotide change appears approximately in 1 every 1000 nucleotides. Length polymorphisms represent more extensive changes in the DNA sequence and approximately are the remaining 10% of polymorphic variability in our genomes.

The NCBI SNP database (www.ncbi.nlm.nih.gov/snp) contains all the SNPs described, arranged by their Reference number, which names all SNPs starting with the letters "rs", followed by a number code, but also including some classical names that had already been given to some SNPs. By clicking on a SNP code, one can get more information and several links, one of them is called "diversity" and shows the different allele frequencies found depending on the study and especially, depending on the sample's ethnicity. There are polymorphic sites with allelic frequencies quite well conserved amongst different ethnicities, but others have relevant differences and we must always pay attention to this point.

The exact biological difference in meaning between "polymorphism" and "mutation" is not always clearly defined. The term "mutation" is classically associated with pathological significance, while "polymorphism" usually refers to a genetic change without health consequences. The problem is that "polymorphism" has also been employed to describe mostly any newly described genetic variant, without having studied it enough to know if it has a pathological consequence or not. The international research project 1000 genomes (www.1000genomes.org) has been a great effort to sequence the whole genome of a thousand different people, so we are still attending to well quantified frequencies of genetic variants, that in some cases will still be measured in not sufficient people and so, knowing exactly the population frequencies of all our genome variants is still a challenge, moreover due to the fact that the frequencies vary amongst different human ethnicities. In conclusion, we must be cautious when interpreting the term "polymorphism" and not assume that it is just a genetic change without any biological consequences, as it may has not been well characterized yet.

The genetic variants that can influence the behavior of a drug in the body, are mainly related to the interaction of the drug with the receptor/ligand involved in their pharmacological action and/or with the systems involved in its pharmacokinetic process of absorption, distribution, metabolism and excretion. So, transport, metabolism and drug target genes are the three groups of genes whose polymorphisms are of interest in pharmacogenetics. In a very simplistic way, an individual carrying a significant polymorphic variant will suffer from different effects from those suffered by the individuals carrying the "normal" variant at the same polymorphic site, but just in the case of being treated with the particular drug affected by that variant. If that individual is not treated with that drug, he may not manifest any effects related to that polymorphism.

Other relevant concepts to understand pharmacogenetics are Haplotipe and Linkage Disequilibrium (LD). Haplotype refers to those alleles of a chromosome, or part thereof, which are physically close and that tend to be inherited together. In our field, it is especially important that more and more frequently the research is focused not on single SNPs, but on combinations of them, forming haplotypes. Although many research has been simplified, studying SNPs analyzed one by one, the real biological significance of these genetic changes must be seen in the resulting effect of groups of SNPs, since the individual effects of each one can be enhanced, reduced or offset by the effects of others. In addition, the linkage disequilibrium, is the situation in which some alleles are present together in a higher frequency than expected, due to its close location in the chromosomes. This is important in SNPs research, since one can study a SNP that is well know and easy to determine, instead of studying another SNP linked to the first, that is more difficult to assess, and the results can be correlated. For instance, in some cases one SNP, with not known biological significance, is correlated with certain clinical consequence, and after a deeper research it is found that actually that first SNP is in fact in linkage disequilibrium with another SNP, unknown or non studied before, that is directly related to that clinical consequence.

In relation to these concepts, we can now understand that SNPs that have not got a clearly studied functional meaning, for example they do not alter the amino acid sequence or are not regulatory in intronic regions, are usually included in research projects. Maybe these SNPs are linked to others that are not taken into consideration but that do produce a direct effect on the gene product. These studies will be completed when information of LD blocks, provided for instance in public consultation databases as HapMap (www.hapmap.org), would be included. These final integrative approaches require powerful statistical and *in silico* analysis, correlating the large amount of information obtained.

4. Genes and drugs

After understanding the basic concepts, we can now enter the approach to the best known gene-drug relationships. There are currently different reference sources that help us in this welter of information, such as the aforementioned HapMap project, the SNP database of NCBI and, to our knowledge, the best pharmacogenetics website which is the Pharmacogenomics Knowledge Base, PharmGKB (www.pharmgkb.org). This latter website, is a very intuitive way of learning and consulting about gene-drug relationships, by performing searches based on gene, SNP, drug or disease; with research and clinical information, and lots of links to external related sites. There we can find a table of the "well-known drug-gene pharmacogenomics associations" which represents the drugs whose relationship with some polymorphic gene has been clearly defined in the literature and is academically accepted, based on extensive reviews of all available information.

The United States Food and Drug Administration (FDA, www.fda.gov) also publishes a list of drugs where a genetic test is recommended or mandatory for the drug administration, explaining which section of the drug label has the genetic-related information.

DRUG	BIOMARKER	DRUG	BIOMARKER
Abacavir	HLA-B*5701	Irinotecan	UGT1A1
Aripiprazole	CYP2D6	Isosorbide and Hydra-lazine62	NAT1, NAT2
Arsenic Trioxide	PML/RARα	Ivacaftor	CFTR
Atomoxetine	CYP2D6	Lapatinib	Her2/neu
Atorvastatin	LDL receptor	Lenalidomide	Chromosome 5q
Azathioprine	TPMT	Letrozole	ER &/ PgR receptor
Boceprevir	IL28B	Maraviroc	CCR5
Brentuximab Vedotin	CD30	Mercaptopurine	TPMT
Busulfan	Ph Chromosome	Metoprolol	CYP2D6
Capecitabine	DPD	Modafinil	CYP2D6
Carbamazepine	HLA-B*1502	Nilotinib	Ph Chromosome, UGT1A1
Carisoprodol	CYP2C19	Nortriptyline	CYP2D6
Carvedilol	CYP2D6	Omeprazole	CYP2C19
Celecoxib	CYP2C9	Panitumumab	EGFR, KRAS
Cetuximab	EGFR, KRAS	Pantoprazole	CYP2C19
Cevimeline	CYP2D6	Paroxetine	CYP2D6
Chlordiazepoxide and Amitriptyline	CYP2D6	Peginterferon alfa-2b	IL28B
Chloroquine	G6PD	Perphenazine	CYP2D6
Cisplatin	TPMT	Pertuzumab	Her2/neu
Citalopram	CYP2C19, CYP2D6	Phenytoin	HLA-B*1502
Clobazam	CYP2C19	Pimozide	CYP2D6
Clomiphene	Rh genotype	Prasugrel	CYP2C19
Clomipramine	CYP2D6	Pravastatin	ApoE2
Clopidogrel	CYP2C19	Propafenone	CYP2D6
Clozapine	CYP2D6	Propranolol	CYP2D6
Codeine	CYP2D6	Protriptyline	CYP2D6
Crizotinib	ALK	Quinidine	CYP2D6
Dapsone	G6PD	Rabeprazole	CYP2C19
Dasatinib	Ph Chromosome	Rasburicase	G6PD
Denileukin Diftitox	CD25	Rifampin, Isoniazid, and Pyrazinamide	NAT1; NAT2
Desipramine	CYP2D6	Risperidone	CYP2D6
Dexlansoprazole	CYP2C19, CYP1A2	Sodium Phenylacetate and Sodium Benzoate	UCD (NAGS; CPS; ASS; OTC; ASL; ARG)
Dextromethorphan and Quinidine	CYP2D6	Sodium Phenylbutyrate	UCD (NAGS; CPS; ASS; OTC; ASL; ARG)
Diazepam	CYP2C19	Tamoxifen	ER receptor
Doxepin	CYP2D6	Telaprevir	IL28B
Drospirenone and Ethinyl Estradiol	CYP2C19	Terbinafine	CYP2D6
Erlotinib	EGFR	Tetrabenazine	CYP2D6
Esomeprazole	CYP2C19	Thioguanine	TPMT
Everolimus	Her2/neu	Thioridazine	CYP2D6

DRUG	BIOMARKER	DRUG	BIOMARKER
Exemestane	ER &/ PgR receptor	Ticagrelor	CYP2C19
Fluorouracil	DPD	Tolterodine	CYP2D6
Fluoxetine	CYP2D6	Tositumomab	CD20 antigen
Fluoxetine and Olanzapine	CYP2D6	Tramadol and Acetaminophen	CYP2D6
Flurbiprofen	CYP2C9	Trastuzumab	Her2/neu
Fluvoxamine	CYP2D6	Tretinoin	PML/RARα
Fulvestrant	ER receptor	Trimipramine	CYP2D6
Galantamine	CYP2D6	Valproic Acid	UCD (NAGS; CPS; ASS; OTC; ASL; ARG)
Gefitinib	EGFR	Vemurafenib	BRAF
Iloperidone	CYP2D6	Venlafaxine	CYP2D6
Imatinib	C-Kit, Ph Chromosome, PDGFR, FIP1L1-PDGFRα	Voriconazole	CYP2C19
Imipramine	CYP2D6	Warfarin	CYP2C9, VKORC1
Indacaterol	UGT1A1		

Table 1. FDA Pharmacogenomic biomarkers in drug labels (adapted from www.fda.gov)

There is certainly a lot of work done, but there is still much to do. Today, there are many publications and many research articles in the area, and the field is growing exponentially, but most of these studies reflect data from very specific conditions, where sets of patients with convenient features and sometimes far from the clinical reality, where included. It is necessary to validate the actual utility of pharmacogenetics in routine medical practice with serious, well-designed studies [8].

4.1. Genes and drugs in transplantation

In the pharmacogenetics of transplantation, as in other therapeutic areas, three groups of genes specifically involved in the response to immunosuppressive therapy have been identified: the genes encoding drug transporter proteins, inward or outward of the cells; the genes encoding metabolic enzymes involved in drug biotransformation and, finally; those encoding receptors or drug targets. Although the great majority of immunosuppressive drugs are transported and metabolized by a limited set of enzymes which mostly are known genes, the interpretation of the results observed in transplanted patients is complicated in many times. One reason for this is that these patients are highly subjected to polytherapy, and so interactions, both pharma-cokinetic and pharmacodynamic, may have great significance and may condition the response to treatment. Another important aspect to consider when interpreting the observed response is the fact that each patient actually contains two different genetic entities: the donor and the recipient. This phenomenon is particularly relevant when the transplanted organs are the liver or the kidney. In these types of transplantation, it must be considered that the drugs admin-istered to the recipient will be metabolized or excreted by the transplanted organ from the donor. In fact, more and more studies in transplantation pharmacogenetics consider both the donor and recipient genotypes to evaluate the response to treatment [9-12].

Moreover, one of the main problems of pharmacogenetic studies is the difficulty to recruit the number of patients needed to achieve sufficient statistical power and demonstrate conclusively the existence of significant clinically relevant differences according the different genotypes, that is, according to the different alleles or variants of a polymorphic site. This is due to the uneven distribution of allele frequencies in the population, which makes it difficult to collect a large enough number of individuals to study minor genotypes. Furthermore, the distribution of allelic frequencies in some genes varies according to ethnicity so, for instance, the expected frequencies of each allele of a polymorphic site in the Caucasian population are not the same as in the Asian. The expected effects of each allelic variant are presumably the same, but the ease for recruiting different genotype patients is not.

Figure 1 shows, in summary, an integrator scheme with the best known genes encoding transporter proteins and enzymes involved in the metabolism of several drugs commonly used in transplantation.

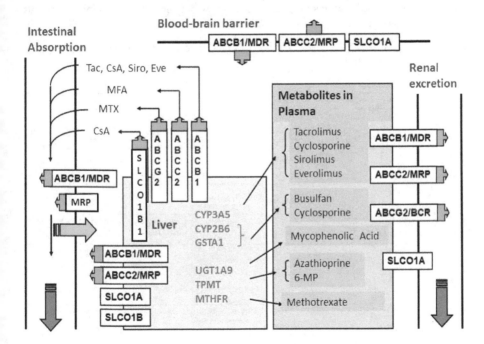

Figure 1. Integrative scheme of pharmacogenetic genes related to transport and metabolism of immunosuppressive drugs for transplantation. (Adapted from ref. 13, ©Astellas Pharma S.A. y Master Line & Prodigio S.L.). The drawing shows a broad view of the location and influence of metabolic enzymes and transporters on the main immunosuppressive drugs used in transplantation. The integrated view of many of the genetic factors that influence the achievement of therapeutic and stationary blood levels, should allow a better interpretation of pharmacogenetic data and also, help improve the safe and effective use of medication.

4.2. Pharmacogenetic examples in renal transplantation

Pharmacogenetic information of immunosuppressants in renal transplantation is mainly related to Tacrolimus, Cyclosporine and Mycophenolic Acid. Sirolimus, Everolimus and Corticoids are also being studied but to a much lesser extent, so we will focus here on the most consolidated conclusion about the first three drugs.

The first two, being both Calcineurin Inhibitors (CNI), share their mechanism of action and so, share transporters, metabolism enzymes and targets and therefore, they also share pharmacogenetic results in most of the cases. The fact that they are both subject of a controlled therapeutic drug monitoring, with "in some way" standardized blood measuring methods, has allowed the publication of many works dealing with correlations between drug levels and polymorphisms [14-23]. To a lesser extent, there are also many works correlating drug adverse effects with SNPs [24-28]. The therapeutic drug monitoring of mycophenolic acid is not as followed as for CNIs, as there is not such a clear consensus about the effects of different blood levels in the possible drug related toxicity. However, many efforts have also been done in the pharmacogenetic studies of this drug [29-36], as it is widely employed in combination with tacrolimus or cyclosporine.

The most consensuated genes regarding polymorphic effects on these three immunosuppressants are shown in table 2.

DRUG	GENE	SNP	Effect
Tacrolimus Cyclosporine	ABCB1 transport	rs1045642 C>T; 3435 C>T	C: higher transporter activity, less drug absorption T: lower transporter activity, more drug absorption
	CYP3A5 metabolism	rs776746 A>G; *1 (A), *3 (G)	Allele *1 carriers have functional enzyme and require higher drug doses to reach target levels. Allele *3 carriers have nonfunctional allele, the enzyme is not metabolizing the drug, so they need lower doses
	CYP3A4 metabolism		Implications not clearly defined
Mycophenolic Acid	UGT1A9 metabolism	-275 T>A -2152 C>T	-275A and -2152T: Increased gene expression, lower exposition to MFA and acute rejection in patients with fixed dose MFA+Tac
	ABCC2 transport	C-24T C3972T	Implications not clearly defined
	IMPDH1 target	rs2278293	Higher risk of leucopenia, lower risk of BPAR
	IMPDH2 target	3757 T>C	C: higher IMPDH activity, higher incidence of BPAR (biopsy-confirmed acute rejection)
	SLCO1B1 transport	*5	Implications not clearly defined

Table 2. Most studied SNPs related to Tacrolimus, Cyclosporine and Mycophenolic Acid in Renal Transplantation.

As shown in the table, even in these SNPs that are the most extensively studied, the clinical implications are not always well established. Many more other SNPs are currently under research consideration, being what we can call "candidates" to have a clinical meaning. Virtually, every polymorphism of a gene implicated in a drug's route of transport, metabolism or mechanism of action is a potential candidate to be investigated. Especially if the polymorphism is known to have a biological consequence on the gene product as for instance, if it is a polymorphism producing a premature STOP codon or a relevant aminoacid change.

Returning to the SNPs in table 2, we will pay attention now to ABCB1 and CYP3A5 most relevant results. In Figure 2, we can see a schematic example of what happens in the intestine epithelial cells, according to the SNP rs1045642 C>T (also known as 3435 C>T) in ABCB1 gene. This gene codes for glicoprotein P (gp-P)which is an adenosine triphosphate-dependent transporter, that pumps many endogenous substances and also xenobiotics, as drugs, outside of the cell. It is specifically expressed in the intestine, liver and kidney, amongst others, and also in several types of leukocytes so it is postulated to function as a protective barrier by actively extruding different compounds out of the cell, into the gut lumen, bile or urine. The expression of ABCB1 in the kidney plays an important role in the renal elimination of metabolic waste products and toxins. It seems like after renal injury, ABCB1 expression is upregulated, which may represent an adpative response in the renal regeneration process [37]. Parallelly, it has been shown that treatment with CNI induces ABCB1 expression both *in vivo* and *in vitro*, which could serve to protect the kidney from the injurious effects of CNIs by facilitating their extrusion. If we add to this, the polymorphic influence shown in figure 2, we can better understand that a failure to adequately upregulate ABCB1 expression or a constitutively low expression in renal cells (as for instance due to 3435 TT variant), could lead to intrarenal accumulation of CNIs and predispose patients to the occurrence of CNI-related nephrotoxicity [38].

Specifically, in renal transplantation, it has been found a correlation between the genotype of donors TT at this SNP and cyclosporine nephrotoxicity [40], while no consistent relationships were found according to the same SNP in the recipient.

Regarding CYP3A5, there is more statistical evidence, especially regarding its impact on CNIs blood levels and these findings have led to some clinical recommendations, as we will see in the next paragraph. Inside the CYP 450 family, the CYP3A subfamily metabolizes more than 50% of all drugs that are currently in use [41]. CYP3A5 is expressed in the small intestine and the liver but also in the kidney.

One of the most relevant studies regarding CYP3A5 SNP rs776746 A>G (*1 (A), *3 (G)) is the one published by Thervet et al. in 2010 [23]. It is a prospective randomized clinical trial that demonstrates the usefulness of this SNP determination before the first tacrolimus dose in renal transplantation. In this study, the pharmacokinetic parameters were correlated with the recipients' genotype and two arms were constructed, one with the classical management of the patients, adjusting tacrolimus doses according to TDM; and the second arm, where the initial dose was chosen according to a previous genetic analysis to include the patients in "CYP3A5 expresser" or "CYP3A5 non-expresser" cathegories. The expressers were given an initial 0.25mg/kg dose and the non-expressers 0.15mg/kg. As a result, the genetically driven dosage was associated with an earlier obtention of tacrolimus concentrations inside the therapeutic range, also with fewer dose adjustments. Also, it was demonstrated that in the first arm, patients with genotype *1 needed double tacrolimus dose to reach the target levels, as compared to those patients that were *3. Moreover, there are also consistent data in pediatric renal transplant recipients [42].

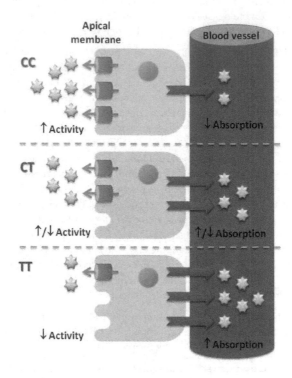

Figure 2. Influence of the functional activity of glycoprotein-P (transporter in apical membrane) in the transport of tacrolimus (green stars) in the intestine epithelium. The diagram shows the different degree of drug absorption due to variations in ABCB1/MDR1 polymorphic site rs1045642. Individuals with TT variant have a decreased transporter activity and hence greater absorption efficiency. CC variant causes more expulsion out of the cell, which decreases absorption. (Figure adapted from ref. 39)

Just as a final remark, we cannot forget to mention the great importance of drug interactions. Although it is not the subject of this chapter, and we are not going to get into it, we just wanted to point here that drug interactions can mask even genetic variations in the clinical practice.

5. Regulatory aspects and final conclusions

5.1. Clinical practice recommendations

We have only seen, with a little bit of detail, two of the SNPs that could actually be influencing the pharmacologic treatment in renal transplantation. And with these two SNPs, only one,

CYP3A5 rs776746, has reached some kind of clinical recommendations. These have not been adopted by any of the regulatory agencies FDA nor EMA, but they already have a strong evidence as to be considered by expert doctors in the area.

The 3rd European Science Foundation- University of Barcelona (ESF-UB) Conference in Biomedicine on Pharmacogenetics and Pharmacogenomics, held in June 2010 in Spain, published a summary of their practical recommendations [43] which include the explained tacrolimus results. They recommend CYP3A5 rs776746 genotyping prior to grafting as it could help to reach steady state plasma tacrolimus concentrations earlier, and therefore prevent overdose (risk of nephrotoxicity) or underdose (risk of acute graft rejection). This recommendation is mainly based on Thervet's publication [23] and suggests the introduction of tacrolimus at 0.15 mg/kg/day when the recpient's genotype is *3/*3, at 0.20 mg/kg/day when it is *3/*1, and at 0.25 mg/kg/day when it is *1/*1; always taking into consideration that the patients will also require the regular TDM.

The Dutch Pharmacogenetics Working Group Guideline from the Royal Dutch Pharmacists Association have also evaluated therapeutic dose recommendations for tacrolimus based on our CYP3A5 SNP [44] and have found evidence to support an interaction between the drug and the gene. However, they do not make dosing recommendations adducing that in dutch transplantation hospitals, the tacrolimus dose is titrated in response to TDM.

5.2. What is a meta-analysis and what is the need of them?

The number of publications is increasing every day in an accelerated manner to limit the ability of researchers and clinicians to assess critically and to assume the results of the studies. This, added to the fact that the knowledge about something is not born due to a single article, but to the integration of many, requires conducting systematic reviews of available evidence, of which there are two types:

- Qualitative systematic reviews, where evidence is presented descriptively

- Quantitative systematic reviews or meta-analyses, which combine the results in a single endpoint and determine the causes of the variations between studies.

Meta-analysis is a summary of different qualitative and quantitative studies (usually randomized controlled trials) that evaluate one aspect whose results are combined using statistic resources to determine the directionality of the effect and the causes of variability between studies. It is the gold standard tool to assess the consistency of an evidence in the effect of a particular intervention, especially when studies are heterogeneous and discordant, when studies evaluating outcomes affect a low number of patients (as it happens when reporting adverse events), when conducting new clinical trials is expensive or when we want to know the existence of patient subgroups responding differently to the intervention analyzed.

- In this way the results allow us to:

- Plan future clinical trials on a related topic.

- Quantify publication bias (as many studies fail to be published because their results are not significant) [45, 46].

- Provide evidence to generate new hypotheses.

- Decide whether further clinical trials are needed on the subject.

- Help to document the approval of the use of interventions by regulatory agents and also expand the knowledge to academics.

Calculate the sample size needed for future clinical trials about a similar topic.

Conducting such studies is cumbersome, it is really time-consuming, requires complex methodological knowledge and its performance is not free of trouble. The main difficulties are the presence of a small number of previously existing studies, the fact that the selected studies to be analysed are usually very heterogeneous and difficult to be combined, and in many of them the necessary information is absent or with low methodological quality. However, meta-analysis studies are low-cost and have high impact.

However, we must be careful as the name "meta-analysis" does not ensure a quality review and readers should critically evaluate it before accepting its results, for which there are currently accessible guides [47, 48]. Its validity largely depends on the quality of the included studies and the absence of bias in its execution [49]. The studies analyzed in the meta-analysis are mostly randomized trials, which are those that offer the best evidence, but there are scenarios where the information comes only from observational studies [50], as studies on etiological hypotheses or adverse events. This represents a challenge as this type of design has a higher risk of bias and lack of essential information for the integration of studies [51]. Furthermore, the inclusion of studies with a large heterogeneity or variability between them, hinders the results interpretation [52], requires the knowledge of statistical tools for proper interpretation [53] and one must know that it is a limitation for the applicability of the results. Meta-analysis is a retrospective process, so it is susceptible to errors of this type of design. It could have biases in any of its stages: in the search and selection of studies, analysis and synthesis of information.

The meta-analysis is the highest level of evidence and summarizes the studies available about a particular matter in a reliable way. Its implementation has its difficulties and limitations, so methodological rigor is required to help reduce the risk of bias and a critical and cautious view of its results.

As far as we know, two meta-analyses have been published regarding clinical implications of CYP3A5 and CNIs in renal transplantation. One is about tacrolimus [54] and its conclusion agrees with the data explained about CYP3A5 expressers/non-expressers dose requirements. The other one deals with cyclosporine [55], and also concludes that there is an association between our SNP and cyclosporine dose-adjusted concentration, where patients carrying *3/*3 genotype will require a lower dose of the drug to reach target levels, compared with *1/*1 or *1/*3 carriers.

5.3. Barriers for the clinical application of Pharmacogenetics

The introduction in the medical practice of new strategies is always difficult, among other reasons due to economic factors and the inertia of much of the professional sector, which is typically conservative. But in the particular case of pharmacogenetics, and genomics in general, there are other social factors that we will now comment, that hinder the implementation of these new techniques.

Contrary to what has usually happened in other fields of biomedicine, in this one we have the paradox that technological progress has gone faster than the advancement of knowledge. Today's technology platforms can just bring in a few days the data that used to take months or even years to achieve. The advances in knowledge of the human genome sequence have been really quick, especially since in February 2001 Nature and Science published simultaneously the results of the Human Genome Project. The enormous progress in data collection through technology could not be accompanied by a corresponding advance in the association of the data with biological effects or implications for medical treatments [56]. A great amount of research investment is still necessary in order to understand and take advantage of this huge avalanche of data.

Clearly, every great discovery is preceded by circumstances that make it possible, and for the deciphering of the human genome, and overall progress of genomics, including Pharmacogenetics-omics, milestones were achieved with the confluence of three fundamental aspects: the opportunity of high performance technologies (high throughput), the multidisciplinary working groups and the development of bioinformatics.

Investment in technology and the big bet of different private companies have been crucial for the rapid performance rate of genetic sequences data collection. In fact, as we have already mentioned, more and more individual human sequences have been obtained, demonstrating the variability of our genome and even small errors in the initial sequencing generations. Anyway, such data cannot give us more information than little white dots on a blackboard, with sometimes very specific information on diseases or even just some predispositions, but little conclusive information for the moment. This is mainly due to two major keys in genetics and biology: the first is that rarely a single gene is responsible for a disease, usually diseases result from the interaction of many genes, with particular variants or defects. The second key is that our phenotype is not an exclusive product of the expression of our genes, instead it is the gene-environment combination. In most cases, the weight of each of the two components in a given disease is difficult to decipher.

Moreover, not only the gene-environment relationship offers serious knowledge gaps, but also the relationships between genes. Everyone knows that life is the result of Systems Biology, waterfalls of activation or repression of components that influence each other. That is the kind of approach that we have to tend to, once we have more experience and results in reductionist studies. Biological systems are complex networks of thousands of routes, many of which are interconnected, biosynthetic pathways, signal transduction pathways, routes of regulating the expression of genes. The integration, representation and modeling of the interconnections of biological information analysis require global, systemic analyses. This is how we enter the era of "omics" referring to global studies, "whole set", where we pass from the analysis of specific phenomena to the search of the interrelationship of phenomena, where we must integrate not only genomics but also proteomics (the sequences and expression patterns of all proteins), metabolomics (identification and quantification of all metabolites) and even transcriptomics (sequences and expression patterns of all transcripts) and to close the circle, reach the interactome (full set of physical interactions between proteins, DNA sequences and RNA). The review of T. Manolio [57] is very useful for understanding the current situation of genomic studies.

In relation to this need for training and knowledge, we will introduce one of the biggest problems facing the Pharmacogenetics and Pharmacogenomics application in our society: as in any area of knowledge that directly affects Health and Drugs, clinical applications arising from Pharmacogenetics should be well regulated and should be given proper use. Both the patient and the doctor must be well informed of the scope and meaning of the data that can be obtained. It is crucial to know what to expect of a pharmacogenetic analysis, realistically, without creating false hopes.

It is said that in a couple of years, the cost for sequencing a complete human genome will be about 1,000$. It is not difficult to imagine that there will soon be many patients who will consult their physicians with their genome sequence in their hand, asking whether they will have cancer or Alzheimer's or not, according to what is written in their genes. Are we prepared to deal with these situations? The New England Journal of Medicine published a series of articles and editorials addressing these issues on the occasion of the first decade of the publication of the human genome, with very interesting articles written by experts in the field, as the great review of Collins and coworkers [58].

And, if we are not prepared for this new tool yet, how will we discriminate between reliable and fraudulent information? Who should be responsible for setting common guidelines to drive us in making decisions about which tests are acceptable and which are not? We think that the key are not only the regulatory agencies, which do not always agree with each other when defining whether a marker is valid or not. However, other agents, Industry, and especially the scientific societies, should be the ones to influence education on these issues and serve as a reference under the most rigorous scientific method.

At the academic level, many efforts have been demanded to these disciplines because they generated great expectations that were not met as fast as expected. Now, regulatory agencies require a greater statistical significance than that of many other types of studies, to accept the validity of a new marker. That is why well designed clinical studies and meta-analyses are necessary for the agencies to accept new validated markers. We must also be aware of the alarm triggered in relation to commercial proposals that are clearly misleading the consumer. Just a quick search on the Internet to realize that they are on sale genotyping chips that offer scientifically implausible predictions, such as predicting vulnerability to sudden death in athletes, obesity, the ability to succeed at school, etc. The U.S. committee SACGHS (the Secretary's Advisory Committee on Genetics, Health and Society) has already issued several reports concerning with the issue and stressing the need to regulate this area of biomedicine in order to not leave the consumer completely unprotected. There are two excellent publications from Dr. JP Evans, illustrating this problem [59, 60].

5.4. The economical impact

Pharmacogenetics must allow not only the money saving through the prevention of a large number of side effects derived from the use of unsuitable drugs, but also it has to reduce the money spending on unnecessary drugs. In the U.S. there is an incidence of adverse effects of 6.2-6.7% of hospitalized patients, representing two million adverse drug reactions per year [61]. Of these, 0.15 to 0.3% are fatal, leading to about 100,000 deaths annually [62]. In Europe, the data are similar.

Today, there are still few studies on the cost-effectiveness of pharmacogenetic studies, although considerable efforts have been made, including regulatory authorities [63-65]. We cannot forget that everyday genotyping platforms are more compact and economical and, as mentioned, even the whole genome sequencing of a patient will have an assumable cost, so it is not difficult to imagine that the benefits will overcome the costs and that the balance will be tilted towards the realization of these studies [66]. A practical example is found in the studies of mutations in the K-ras gene in colorectal cancer patients to decide about treatment with Cetuximab, which are rendering large amounts of data regarding the savings thanks to the genotyping of patients, avoiding ineffective treatment in 40% of cases.

In conclusion, the economical and clinical benefits of pharmacogenetics are day by day, clearly surpassing its costs. We need to have especialized personnel, to help us know how to interpret the pharmacogenetic information, always in close contact with clinicians and research advances. We cannot obviate this new and real tool for the benefit of our patients' health.

Author details

María José Herrero[1*], Virginia Bosó[1], Luis Rojas[1,2], Sergio Bea[3], Jaime Sánchez Plumed[3], Julio Hernández[3], Jose Luis Poveda[4] and Salvador F. Aliño[5]

*Address all correspondence to: maria.jose.herrero@uv.es

1 Unidad de Farmacogenética, Instituto Investigación Sanitaria La Fe, Servicio de Farmacia, Hospital Universitario y Politécnico La Fe, Valencia, Spain

2 Hospital clínico de la Pontificia Universidad Católica de Chile, Dpto. Medicina Interna, y Centro de Investigaciones Clínicas, Chile

3 Servicio Nefrología, Hospital Universitario y Politécnico La Fe, Valencia, Spain

4 Servicio de Farmacia, Hospital Universitario y Politécnico La Fe, Valencia, Spain

5 Unidad Farmacología Clínica, Hospital Universitario y Politécnico La Fe; Dpto. Farmacología, Fac. Medicina, Universidad de Valencia, Valencia, Spain

References

[1] Herrero, M. J, Marqués, M. R, Sánchez-plumed, J, Prieto, M, Almenar, L, Pastor, A, Galán, J. B, Poveda, J. L, & Aliño, S. F. Farmacogenética/ Farmacogenómica en el trasplante. In: Roche. Bases para la atención farmacéutica al paciente trasplantado. Madrid: (2009). , 331-341.

[2] Aliño, S. F, Herrero, M. J, & Poveda, J. L. De la población al paciente: diferencias individuales en la respuesta a los medicamentos. In: López E., Poveda JL. editors. Evaluación y selección de medicamentos basadas en la evidencia. Madrid: (2008). , 259-282.

[3] Hardy, J, & Singleton, A. Genomewide association studies and human disease. New England Journal of Medicine (2009). , 360, 1759-68.

[4] Herrero, M. J, Aliño, S. F, Poveda, J. L, et al. Farmacogenética: una realidad clínica.., Madrid: Astellas Pharma- Master Line Ed; (2010).

[5] EMEA/CHMP/ICH/437986/(2006). Definitions for genomic biomarkers, pharmacogenomics, pharmacogenetics, genomic data and sample coding categories. www.ema.europa.eu/accessed 20 June 2012)

[6] Aliño, S. F, Dasí, F, & Herrero, M. J. Farmacogenómica y terapia génica en el trasplante.In: Edipharma. Bases para la atención farmacéutica al paciente transplantado, (2006). , 305-316.

[7] Drews, J. Genomic sciences and the medicine of tomorrow. Nat. Biotechnol (1996). , 11, 1516-1518.

[8] Daly, A. K. Pharmacogenetics and human genetic polymorphisms. Biochem. J. (2010). , 429, 435-449.

[9] Provenzani, A, et al. The effect of CYP3A5 and ABCB1 single nucleotide polymorphisms on tacrolimus dose requirements in Caucasian liver transplant patients. Ann Transplant (2009). , 14, 23-31.

[10] Herrero, M. J, Almenar, L, Jordán, C, Sánchez, I, Poveda, J. L, & Aliño, S. F. Clinical interest of pharmacogenetic polymorphisms in the immunosupressive treatment after heart transplantation. Transplantation Proceedings (2010). , 42, 3181-3182.

[11] Herrero, M. J, Sánchez-plumed, J, Galiana, M, Bea, S, Marqués, M. R, & Aliño, S. F. Influence of the pharmacogenetic polymorphisms in the routine immunosuppression therapy after renal transplantation. Transplantation Proceedings (2010). , 42, 3134-3136.

[12] Ran Jun KLee W., Jang M., et al. Tacrolimus concentrations in relations to CYP3A and ABCB1 polymorphisms in solid organ transplant recipients in Korea. Transplantation (2009). , 87, 1225-1231.

[13] Herrero, M. J, Poveda, J. L, García, P, & Aliño, S. F. Metodología, retos y puntos débiles en la aplicación de la Farmacogenética. Madrid: Ergon; (2011).

[14] Anglicheau et alAssociation of MDR1 polymorphism with the tacrolimus dose requirements in renal transplant recipients. J. Am. Soc Nephrol. (2003). , 14(7), 1889-96.

[15] Bouamar, R, Hesselink, D. A, Van Schaik, R. H, Weimar, W, Macphee, I. A, De Fijter, J. W, & Van Gelder, T. Polymorphisms in CYP3A5, CYP3A4, and ABCB1 are not associated with cyclosporine pharmacokinetics nor with cyclosporine clinical end points after renal transplantation. Ther Drug Monit. (2011). , 33(2), 178-184.

[16] Haufroid, V, et al. The effect of CYP3A5 and MDR1 (ABCB1) polymorphism on CYA and Tacrolimus dose requirements and trough blood level in stable renal transplant patients. Pharmacogenetics (2004). , 14, 147-154.

[17] Goto, M, et al. CYP3A5*1-carrying graft liver reduces the concentration/oral dose ratio of tacrolimus in recipients of living-donor liver transplantation. Pharmacogenetics (2004). , 14, 471-478.

[18] Thervet, E, et al. Impact of CYP3A5 genetic polymorphism on TC doses and concentration to dose ratio in renal trasplant recipients. Transplantation (2003).

[19] Zheng, H, et al. Tacrolimus dosing in adult lung transplant patients is related to CYP3A5 gen polymorphisms. Am J. Transplant. (2003). , 3, 477-483.

[20] MacPhee IAet al. Tacrolimus pharmacogenetics polimorphism associated with expression of CYP3A5 and Gly-P correlate with dose requirement. Transplantation (2002). , 74(11), 1486-1489.

[21] MacPhee IAet al. The influence of pharmacogenetics on the time to achieve target tacrolimus concentration after kidney transplantation. Am J. Transplant. (2004). , 4, 914-919.

[22] Haufroid, V, et al. CYP3A5 and MDR1 (ABCB1) polymorphism and tacrolimus pharmacokinetics in renal transplant candidates: guidelines from an experimental study. Am J. Transplant. (2006). , 6, 2706-2713.

[23] Thervet, E, Loriot, M. A, Barbier, S, et al. Optimization of initial tacrolimus dose using pharmacogenetic testing. Clin Pharmacol Ther (2010). , 87(6), 721-726.

[24] Undre, N. A, et al. Low systemic exposure to tacrolimus correlates with acute rejection. Trasplant. Prc. (1999). , 31, 296-298.

[25] Yamauchi, A, et al. Neurotoxicity induced by tacrolimus after liver transplantation: relation to genetic polimorphism of the ABCB1 (MDR1) gene. Trasplantation (2002). , 74, 571-572.

[26] Zheng et alTacrolimus nephrotoxicity is predicted by MDR1 exon 21 polimorphism whereas dosing is predicted by CYP3A5 polimorphism in adult lung transplant patients. American Transplant Congress, Washington DC. Transplantation (2003).

[27] Kuypers et alCYP3A5 and CYP3A4 but not MDR1 polimorphism determine longterm Tacrolimus disposition and drug-related nephrotoxicity in renal recipients. Clin Pharmacol Ther (2007). , 82(6), 711-25.

[28] Glowacki, F, Lionet, A, Buob, D, Labalette, M, Allorge, D, Provo, t F, Hazzan, M, Noe, l C, Broly, F, Cauffiez, C, & Cyp, A. and ABCB1 polymorphisms in donor and recipient: impact on Tacrolimus dose requirements and clinical outcome after renal transplantation. Nephrol Dial Transplant. (2011). , 26, 3046-3050.

[29] Lloberas et alInfluence of MRP2 on MPA pharmacokinetics in renal transplant recipients-results of the Pharmacogenomic Substudy within the Symphony Study. Nephrol Dial Transplant (2011). , 26(11), 3784-3793.

[30] Michellon, H, et al. SLCO1B1 genetic polymorphism influences mycophenolic acid tolerance in renal tranplant recipients. Pharmacogenomics (2010). , 11(12), 1703-1713.

[31] Picard, N. Wah Yee S., Woillard JB., Lebranchu Y., Le Meur Y., Giacomini KM., Marquet P. The role of organic anion-transporting polypeptides and their common genetic variants in mycophenolic acid pharmacokinetics. Clin Pharmacol Ther. (2010). , 87(1), 100-108.

[32] Kagaya, H, Miura, M, Saito, M, Habuchi, T, & Satoh, S. Correlation of IMPDH1 gene polymorphisms with subclinical acute rejection and mycophenolic acid exposure parameters on day 28 after renal transplantation. Basic Clin Pharmacol Toxicol. (2010). , 107(2), 631-636.

[33] Sánchez-fructuoso, A. I, Maestro, M. L, Calvo, N, Viudarreta, M, Pérez-flores, I, Veganzone, S, De La Orden, V, Ortega, D, Arroyo, M, & Barrientos, A. The prevalence of uridine diphosphate-glucuronosyltransferase 1A9 (UGT1A9) gene promoter region single-nucleotide polymorphisms T-275A and C-2152T and its influence on mycophenolic acid pharmacokinetics in stable renal transplant patients. Transplantation Proceedings (2009). , 41, 2313-2316.

[34] Johnson, L'A. A, Oetting, W. S, Basu, S, Prausa, S, Matas, A, & Jacobson, P. A. Pharmacogenetic effect of the UGT polymorphismson mycophenolate is modified by calcineurin inhibitors. Eur J Clin Pharmacol (2008). , 64, 1047-1056.

[35] Miura, M, Satoh, S, Inoue, K, Kagaya, H, Saito, M, Inoue, T, Suzuki, T, & Habuchi, T. Influence of SLCO1B1, 1B3, 2B1 and ABCC2 genetic polymorphisms on mycophenolic acid pharmacokinetics in Japanese renal transplant recipients. Eur J Clin Pharmacol (2007). , 63, 1161-1169.

[36] van Schaik RHN. et alUGT1A9-275T>A/-2152 C>T polymorphisms correlate with low MPA exposure and acute rejection in MMF/Tacrolimus-treated kidney transplant patients. Clinical Phramacology and Therapeutics (2009). , 86(3), 319-27.

[37] Huls, M. van den Heuvel JJMW., Dijkman HBPM., et al. ABC transporter expression profiling after ischemic reperfusion injury in mouse kidney. Kidney Int. (2006). , 69, 2186-2193.

[38] Hesselink, D. A, Bouamar, R, & Van Gelder, T. The pharmacogenetics of calcineurin inhibitor-related nephrotoxicity. Ther Drug Monit. (2010). , 32(4), 387-393.

[39] Galiana, M, Herrero, M. J, Bosó, V, Bea, S, Ros, E, Sánchez-plumed, J, Poveda, J. L, & Aliño, S. F. Pharmacogenetics of immunosuppressive drugs in renal transplantation. In: Long L, editor. Renal Transplantation- Updates and Advances, Rijeka: InTech; (2012). , 143-162.

[40] Hauser, I. A, Schaeffeler, E, Gauer, S, et al. ABCB1 genotype of the donor but not of the recipient is a major risk factor for cyclosporine-related nephrotoxicity after renal transplantation. J Am Soc Nephrol. (2005). , 16, 1501-1511.

[41] Evans, W. E, & Mcleod, H. L. Pharmacogenomics: drug disposition, drug targets, and side effects. N Engl J Med. (2003). , 348, 538-549.

[42] Zhao, W, Elie, V, Roussey, G, et al. Population pharmacokinetics and pharmacogenetics of tacrolimus in de novo pediatric kidney transplant recipients. Clin Pharmacol Ther (2009). , 86(6), 609-618.

[43] Becquemont, L, Alfirevic, A, Amstutz, U, et al. Practical recommendations for phar-macogenomics-based prescription: 2010 ESF-UB conference on pharmacogenetics and pharmacogenomics. Pharmacogenomics (2011).

[44] Swen, J. J, Nijenhuis, M, De Boer, A, et al. Pharmacogenetics: from bench to byte-an update of guidelines. Clinical Pharmacology and Therapeutics (2011). , 89(5), 662-673.

[45] Montori, V. M, Smieja, M, & Guyatt, G. H. Publication bias: a brief review for clinicians. Mayo Clin Proc (2000). , 75(12), 1284-1288.

[46] Egger, M, & Smith, G. D. Bias in location and selection of studies. BMJ (1998). , 316(7124), 61-66.

[47] Liberati, A, Altman, D. G, Tetzlaff, J, Mulrow, C, Gotzsche, P. C, Ioannidis, J. P, et al. The PRISMA statement for reporting systematic reviews and meta-analyses of studies that evaluate healthcare interventions: explanation and elaboration. BMJ (2009). b2700.

[48] Shuster, J. J. Review: Cochrane handbook for systematic reviews for interventions, Version 5.1.0, published 3/2011. Julian P.T. Higgins and Sally Green, Editors. Research Synthesis Methods (2011). , 2(2), 126-130.

[49] Simon, R. Meta-analysis of clinical trials: opportunities and limitations. In: Stangl D, Berry D, editors. Meta-Analysis in Medicine and Health Policy New York; (2000).

[50] Berlin, J. A. Invited Commentary: Benefits of Heterogeneity in Meta-analysis of Data from Epidemiologic Studies. American Journal of Epidemiology (1995). , 142(4), 383-387.

[51] Blettner, M, Sauerbrei, W, Schlehofer, B, Scheuchenpflug, T, & Friedenreich, C. Traditional reviews, meta-analyses and pooled analyses in epidemiology. Int J Epidemiol (1999). , 28(1), 1-9.

[52] Altman, D. G. Matthews JNS. Statistics Notes: Interaction 1: heterogeneity of effects. BMJ (1996).

[53] Higgins, J. P, & Thompson, S. G. Quantifying heterogeneity in a meta-analysis. Stat Med (2002). , 21(11), 1539-1558.

[54] Tang, H. L, Xie, H. G, Yao, Y, & Hu, Y. F. Lower tacrolimus daily dose requirements and acute rejection rates in the CYP3A5 nonexpressers than expressers. Pharmacogenetics and Genomics (2011). , 21, 713-720.

[55] Zhu, H. J, Yuan, S. H, Fang, Y, Sun, X. Z, Kong, H, & Ge, W. H. The effect of CYP3A5 polymorphism on dose-adjusted cyclosporine concentration in renal transplant recipients: a meta-analysis. The Pharmacogenomics Journal (2011). , 11, 237-246.

[56] Varmus, H. Ten years on- the human genome and medicine. N Engl J Med (2010). , 362, 2028-29.

[57] Manolio, T. A. Genomewide association studies and assessment of the risk of disease. N Engl J Med (2010). , 363, 166-176.

[58] Feero, W. G, Guttmacher, A. E, & Collins, F. S. Genomic medicine-an updated primer. N Engl J Med (2010). , 362, 2001-2011.

[59] Evans, J. P, & Green, R. C. Direct to consumer genetic testing: avoiding a culture war. Genet Med (2009). , 11, 568-569.

[60] Evans, J. P, Dale, D. C, & Fomous, C. Preparing for a consumer-driven genomic age. N Engl J Med. (2010). , 363(12), 1099-1103.

[61] Pirmohamed, M, James, S, et al. Adverse drug reactions as cause of admission to hospital: prospective analysis of 18820 patients. Br Med J (2004). , 329, 15-19.

[62] Evans, W. E, & Relling, M. V. Moving towards individualized medicine with pharmacogenomics. Nature (2004). , 429, 646-68.

[63] Ibarreta, D, et al. Cost-effectiveness of pharmacogenomics in clinical practice: a case study of thiopurine methyltransferase genotyping in acute lymphoblastic leukemia in Europe. Pharmacogenomics (2006). , 7, 783-92.

[64] Woelderink, A, Ibarreta, D, Hopkins, M. M, & Rodriguez-cerezo, E. The current clinical practice of pharmacogenetic testing in Europe: TPMT and HER2 as case studies. Pharmacogenomics J (2006). , 6, 3-7.

[65] Hopkins, M. M, Ibarreta, D, Gaisser, S, et al. Putting pharmacogenetics into practice. Nature Biotechnology (2006). , 24, 403-410.

[66] Sheffield, L. J, & Phillimore, H. E. Clinical use of pharmacogenomic tests in (2009). Clin Biochem Rev 2009; , 30, 55.

Chapter 10

Clinical Pharmacology and Therapeutic Drug Monitoring of Immunosuppressive Agents

Ana Luisa Robles Piedras,
Minarda De la O Arciniega and
Josefina Reynoso Vázquez

Additional information is available at the end of the chapter

1. Introduction

Immunosuppressive drugs are used to reduce the immune response in organ transplantation and autoimmune disease. In transplantation, the major classes of immunosuppressive drugs used today are: (1) glucocorticoids, (2) calcineurin inhibitors, (3) antiproliferative/antimetabolic agents, and (4) biologics (antibodies). These drugs have met with a high degree of clinical success in treating conditions such as acute immune rejection of organ transplants and severe autoimmune diseases. However, such therapies require lifelong use and nonspecifically suppress the entire immune system, exposing patients to considerably higher risks of adverse effects [1].

The pharmacokinetics of the immunosuppressive drugs is complex and unpredictable. A narrow therapeutic index unique to each patient, as well as variable absorption, distribution, and elimination, are characteristics of these drugs. Therapeutic drug monitoring plays a key role in helping clinicians maintain blood and plasma levels of immunosuppressive drugs within their respective therapeutic ranges. Variation in concentrations outside the narrow therapeutic ranges can result in adverse clinical outcomes. Therapeutic drug monitoring ensures that concentrations are not too high or too low, thereby reducing the risks of toxicity or rejection, respectively. This chapter briefly reviews some immunosuppressive drugs: cyclosporine, tacrolimus, mycophenolic acid, sirolimus, everolimus, azathioprine, daclizumab and basiliximab, alemtuzumab and glucocorticoids. A general discussion of mechanism of action and side effects of these immunosuppressive agents used more commonly today are described below, followed by an overview of general principles of therapeutic drug monitoring and concluding with brief information about monitoring of individual immunosuppressive agents as well as a brief description of future trends in immunosuppression therapy.

2. Mechanism of action and side effects

2.1. Cyclosporine A (CsA)

CsA is a cyclic polypeptide immunosuppressant consisting of 11 amino acids. It is produced as a metabolite of the fungus species *Tolypocladium inflatum* Gams. CsA generally is recognized as the agent that ushered in the modern era of organ transplantation, increasing the rates of early engraftment, extending kidney graft survival, and making cardiac and liver transplantation possible. Clinical indications for CsA are kidney, liver, heart, and other organ transplantation; rheumatoid arthritis; and psoriasis. The dose of CsA varies, depending on the organ transplanted and the other drugs used in the specific treatment protocols. Dosage is guided by signs of rejection (too low a dose), renal or other toxicity (too high a dose), and close monitoring of blood levels [1].

2.1.1. Mechanism of action

CsA suppresses some humoral immunity, but is more effective against T-cell-dependent immune mechanisms such as those underlying transplant rejection and some forms of autoimmunity. Its actions appear to be dependent upon binding to intracellular sites of action. Because of its high lipophilicity, CsA enters cells easily to gain access to the site of action [1]. The intracellular protein most closely linked to the immunosuppressive activity of CsA is cyclophilin. CsA forms a complex with cyclophilin, a cytoplasmic receptor protein present in target cells. This complex binds to calcineurin to block its phosphatase activity (Table 1). Calcineurin-catalyzed dephosphorylation is required for movement of a component of the nuclear factor of activated T lymphocytes (NFAT) into the nucleus. Calcineurin phosphatase activity is inhibited after physical interaction with the cyclosporine/cyclophilin complex. This prevents Ca^{2+}-stimulated dephosphorylation of the cytosolic component of NFAT such that NFAT does not enter the nucleus, gene transcription is not activated, and the T lymphocyte fails to respond to specific antigenic stimulation. By binding to cyclophilin, the antigenic response of helper T lymphocytes is inhibited; the production of interleukin-2 and interferon-gamma is suppressed [2-3]. In addition, production of the receptor site for interleukin-2 on T lymphocytes is inhibited by CsA and also increases expression of transforming growth factor-β (TGF-β), a potent inhibitor of IL-2–stimulated Tcell proliferation and generation of cytotoxic T lymphocytes (CTL) [4-8].

2.1.2. Side effects

The principal side effects to CsA therapy are hypertension, nephrotoxicity, tremor, hirsutism, hyperlipidemia, nausea and vomiting, gingival hyperplasia, and hepatotoxicity [1,9]. Hypertension is a common adverse effect of CsA, with the incidence decreasing over time. Generally, mild to moderate hypertension may occur in approximately 50% of renal transplant patients and most cardiac transplant patients. In liver transplant patients (n=75), 27% experienced hypertension. Incidence: 13% to 53% [9]. Discontinuation of CsA therapy may be required for persistent blood pressure elevation despite adjustments in therapy. Antihypertensive agents such as calcium-channel blockers may be used, with isradipine and nifedipine most appropriate since they do not interfere with CsA metabolism. Other calcium-channel blockers (eg, diltiazem and verapamil) may increase cyclosporine levels. Patients with preexisting hypertension controlled by beta-blockers may continue to receive the same therapy. Angiotensin converting enzyme inhibitors and diuretics are not recommended [10]. Probable mechanisms for cyclosporine induced hypertension involve increased prostaglandin synthesis, decreased free water excretion, and decreased sodium and potassium excretion [11]. CsA is nephrotoxic, the mechanism by which CsA causes nephrotoxicity is attributed to changes in vasomotor tone induced by activation of the sympathetic nervous system [12]. Tremor was reported to appear within a few days of initiating CsA therapy and was considered dose dependent. Incidence: 12% to 55% [9].

Immunosuppressive agent	Site of Action
Cyclosporine and tacrolimus	Calcineurin (inhibits phosphatase activity)
Mycophenolic acid	Inosine monophosphate dehydrogenase (inhibits activity)
Sirolimus and everolimus	Protein kinase involved in cellcycle progression (mTOR) (inhibits activity)
Azathioprine	Deoxyribonucleic acid (false nucleotide incorporation)
Daclizumab and basiliximab	IL-2 receptor (block IL-2–mediated T-cell activation)
Alemtuzumab	Cell surface glycoprotein CD52
Glucocorticoids	Glucocorticoid response elements in DNA (regulate gene transcription)

Table 1. Sites of action of immunosuppressive agents on T-cell activation [1]

Administration of CsA adversely affects plasma lipoprotein and cholesterol levels causing hyperlipidemia [9]. In a study CsA increased total cholesterol by 21%, low-density lipoproteins by 31%, and apolipoproteins by 12% over 27 days [13]. Gingival hyperplasia was reported in 4% to 16% of patients treated with CsA [9]. Histologically, CsA-induced gingival overgrowth is characterized by cellular hyperplasia along with myxomatous changes and accumulation of collagen [14]. Reduction of the dose of CsA may result in complete resolution of gingival hyperplasia [15,16].

2.2. Tacrolimus (TRL)

TRL (Prograf®) is a macrolide antibiotic produced by *Streptomyces tsukubaensis*. It is practically insoluble in water. TRL is indicated for the prophylaxis of solid-organ allograft rejection in a manner similar to CsA. The recommended starting dose for TRL injection is 0.03 to 0.05 mg/kg per day as a continuous infusion. Recommended initial oral doses are 0.15 to 0.2 mg/kg per day for adult kidney transplant patients, in two divided doses 12 hours apart. These dosages are intended to achieve typical blood trough levels in the 5 to 15 ng/mL range. Pediatric patients generally require higher doses than do adults [1,17].

2.2.1. Mechanism of action

The compound is chemically distinct from CsA but both agents elicit similar immunosuppressant effects. TRL suppresses both humoral (antibody) and cell-mediated immune responses. Like CsA, TRL inhibits Tcell activation by inhibiting calcineurin [17]. The proposed mechanism for this effect is binding to an intracellular protein FK506-binding protein–12 (FKBP-12), immunophilin structurally related to cyclophilin. A complex of tacrolimus-FKBP-12, Ca2+, calmodulin, and calcineurin then forms, which inhibits the phosphatase activity of calcineurin (Table 1). As described for CsA the inhibition of phosphatase activity prevents dephosphorylation and nuclear translocation of NFAT and inhibits T-cell activation. Thus, although the intracellular receptors differ, CsA and TRL target the same pathway for immunosuppression [1,18]. The immunosuppressive activity of TRL is, however, more marked than that of CsA. Studies on cultured CD4+ (T-helper) lymphocytes have demonstrated that TRL is at least 100 times more potent than CsA (weight basis) in selectively inhibiting secretion of various cytokines (i.e., interleukin-2, interleukin-3, interferon-gamma) [19,20]. The action of TRL on lymphocytes is more difficult to reverse than that of CsA; this may be attributable to the effect of TRL on impairing the expression of interleukin-2 receptors on alloantigen-stimulated T-cells [19]. TRL possesses another important effect in addition to the inhibition of IL-2 gene transcription, to be exact the ability to act as a general inhibitor of the protein secretory pathway, which strongly suggests that the diabetogenic effect of the TRL could be caused by the blockade of insulin secretion. This novel effect also provides an explanation for other side-effects observed in immunosuppressive treatment [1,21,22].

2.2.2. Side effects

TRL is an established immunosuppressant for the prevention and treatment of allograft rejection in organ transplantation. However, TRL therapy also has several adverse effects like nephrotoxicity, hypertension, hyperkalemia, hyperglycemia, hyperlipidemia, neurotoxicity (tremor, headache, dizziness, seizure), gastrointestinal complaints, and diabetes are all associated with TRL use [18].

Nephrotoxicity has been reported with TRL therapy, particularly when used in high doses. Incidence: 36% to 59% [23]. Acute nephrotoxicity is characterized by an increased serum creatinine and/or a decrease in urine output, and is generally reversible. Chronic nephrotoxicity is associated with increased serum creatinine, decreased kidney graft life, and characteristic histologic changes observed on renal biopsy; these changes are usually progressive. Renal function should be monitored closely [23,24]. In systemic formulations hypertension occurred in 13% to 89% of patients receiving TRL in clinical trials. Antihypertensive therapy may be required. Potassium sparing diuretics, ACE inhibitors, and angiotensin receptor blockers should be used with careful consideration since due to the potential to cause hyperkalemia. Calcium channel blockers may be effective in treating TRL associated hypertension, but caution is warranted since interference with TRL metabolism may require a dosage reduction. [23,25]. Hyperlipidemia was reported as one of the more common adverse events in TRL-treated heart transplant recipients. Incidence: 10% to 34% [23]. In clinical trials tremor has occurred in 15% to 56% of patients receiving TRL [23,26]. In systemic formulations headache occurred in 24% to 64% of patients receiving TRL in clinical trials. Headache may respond to a dosage reduction [23]. In clinical trials hyperglycemia occurred in 21% to 70% of patients receiving TRL [23]. New onset diabetes mellitus has been reported in kidney, liver, and heart transplant patients receiving TRL therapy. Incidence: 11% to 22%. Close monitoring of blood glucose concentrations is recommended [23,27].

2.3. Mycophenolic acid (MPA)

MPA is a secondary metabolite produced by *Penicillium brevicompactum*, which has antibiotic and immunosuppressive properties used to prevent rejection of solid organ transplants [28]. It is highly soluble in aqueous media at physiological pH. The drug is marketed as the ester prodrug mycophenolate mofetil (CellCept®) (MMF) for kidney, liver, and heart transplants or enteric-coated mycophenolate sodium (Myfortic®) for kidney transplants [1,29].

2.3.1. Mechanism of action

MPA produces potent selective, noncompetitive, and reversible inhibition of inosine mono-phosphate dehydrogenase (IMPDH), an important enzyme in the *de novo* pathway of guanine nucleotide synthesis (Table 1). B and T lymphocytes are highly dependent on this pathway for cell proliferation, while other cell types can use salvage pathways; MPA therefore selectively inhibits lymphocyte proliferation and functions, including antibody formation, cellular adhesion, and migration [1,30]. *In vitro* and *in vivo* studies have demonstrated the ability of MPA to block proliferative responses of T and B lymphocytes, and inhibit antibody formation and the generation of cytotoxic T-cells [31]. In a preclinical study in mice, MPA increased survival of heart and pancreatic islet cell allografts. Studies in rats have also demonstrated prolonged heart allograft survival, as well as reversal of acute rejection and prevention of rejection in the sensitized animal. Antirejection effects have been attributed to decreased recruitment of activated lymphocytes to the graft site [32].

2.3.2. Side effects

The principal adverse effects of MPA are gastrointestinal, these include diarrhea, nausea and vomiting; hypertension; hematologic effects (anemia and leukopenia) and neurologic effects (anxiety asthenia dizziness headache insomnia tremor). There also is an increased incidence of some infections, especially sepsis associated with cytomegalovirus [1,33-35]. Diarrhea was reported in 36.1% of renal transplant patients, 45.3% of cardiac transplant patients, and 51.3% of hepatic transplant patients in a clinical study. Vomiting was reported in 33.9% of cardiac transplant patients, and 32.9% of hepatic transplant patients. Nausea was reported in 23.6% of renal transplant patients, 54% of cardiac transplant patients, and 54.5% of hepatic transplant. The incidence of adverse gastrointestinal complications requiring dose reduction. Usually occurs early in therapy and respond to dose reduction or switching from two to three divided daily doses [34].

Hypertension was reported in 28.2% of renal transplant patients, 77.5% of cardiac transplant patients, and 62.1% of hepatic transplant patients [34]. Leukopenia was 23.2% and 34.5% in renal transplant, 30.4% in cardiac transplant, and 45.8% in hepatic transplant in a clinical study. Complete blood counts should be performed weekly during the first month, twice monthly for the second and third months of treatment, then monthly through the first year [34].

2.4. Sirolimus (SRL) and Everolimus (EVL)

SRL(also known as Rapamycin and Rapamune®) is a macrocyclic lactone produced by the actinomycete *Streptomyces hygroscopicus*, with immunosuppressive, antitumor, and antifungal properties. SRL appears to be synergistic with CsA in kidney transplantation, but with a different side-effect profile. It is an immunosuppressive agent of potential benefit in clinical liver transplantation. EVL is an analogue of SRL with immunosuppressive and antiproliferative activity. It is closely related chemically and clinically to SRL but has distinct pharmacokinetics. The main difference is a shorter half-life and thus a shorter time to achieve steady state concentrations of the drug [1,36].

2.4.1. Mechanism of action of SRL

SRL has been demonstrated to block the response of T- and B-cell activation by cytokines, which prevents cell-cycle progression and proliferation. Intracellularly, sirolimus forms a complex with cytosolic FK-binding proteins, primarily FKBP-12, considered essential for functionality; however, the sirolimus–FKBP-12 complex does not affect calcineurin activity. It binds to and inhibits a protein kinase, designated mammalian target of rapamycin (mTOR) (Table 1), which is a key enzyme in cell-cycle progression. Inhibition of mTOR blocks cell-cycle progression at the G1 to S phase transition [37,38]. Specific biochemical steps inhibited by SRL include activation of p70S6 kinase, activation of the cdk2/cyclinE complex, and phosphorylation of retinoblastoma protein [37,38]. SRL appears to be less nephrotoxic than CsA and TRL; this may be related to its lack of effect on calcineurin [1,38]. In preclinical studies (*in vitro* and *in vivo*), additive or synergistic immunosuppressive effects were observed when SRL was combined with TRL, CsA, MMF, and brequinar [37].

2.4.2. Side effects of SRL

The use of SRL in renal transplant patients is associated with a dose-dependent increase in serum cholesterol and triglycerides that may require treatment. Other studies have identified hyperlipidemia and thrombocytopenia as significant SRL side effects [39]. In the other hand, while immunotherapy with SRL *per se* is not nephrotoxic, patients treated with CsA plus SRL have impaired renal function compared to patients treated with CsA and either azathioprine or placebo. Renal function therefore must be monitored closely in such patients. Other adverse effects include anemia, leukopenia, thrombocytopenia, hypokalemia or hyperkalemia, fever, and gastrointestinal effects. Delayed wound healing may occur with SRL use. As with other immunosuppressive agents, there is an increased risk of neoplasms, especially lymphomas, and infections [1,36,37].

2.4.3. Mechanism of action of EVL

Like SRL, EVL binds to the cytosolic immunophyllin FKBP12; both agents inhibit growth factor-driven cell proliferation, including that of T-cells and vascular smooth muscle cells. After binding to and forming a complex with the cytoplasmic protein FKBP-12, this complex binds to and inhibits the mammalian Target Of Rapamycin (mTOR) and phosphorylates P70 S6 ribosomal protein kinase (a substrate of mTOR) (Table 1). The phosphorylation of P70 S6 ribosomal protein kinase by the EVL complex prevents protein synthesis and cell proliferation. The EVL:FKBP-12 complex does not affect calcineurin activity [40,41]. Binding of EVL to FKBP12 is weaker than that of SRL (about 3-fold), related to 40-O-alkylation, and this correlates with a 2- to 3-fold lower in vitro immunosuppressive activity for EVL. However, the oral *in vivo* activity of EVL has been at least equipotent to oral SRL in several animal allotransplantation/autoimmune disease models. This appears related to the chemical modification in EVL (2-hydroxyethyl chain), providing more favorable pharmacokinetic properties (eg, absorption, disposition) which compensate for relatively poor *in vitro* activity [40]. EVL and SRL antagonize TRL based calcineurin inhibition via saturation of FKBP12 [1,42].

2.4.4. Side effects of EVL

Side effects seem to be the same as with SRL [1]. Endocrine abnormalities, including hyperlipidemia and hypertriglyceridemia, have been reported with EVL treatment. Monitoring for hyperlipidemia is recommended in all patients; diet, exercise, and lipid lowering therapy should be initiated if hyperlipidemia occurs. In a clinical study with EVL, the most important causes of discontinuation in 69 patients were severe infections (2.3%), pneumonitis (6.8 %), acute rejection episode (4.1%), proteinuria (4.1%). Although the overall incidence discontinuation due to side effects was higher in the EVL than SRL group, there was no greater frequency of severe side effects [43,44].

2.5. Azathioprine

Azathioprine is a purine antimetabolite. It is an imidazolyl derivative of 6-mercaptopurine. Azathioprine was first introduced as an immunosuppressive agent in 1961, helping to make allogeneic kidney transplantation possible. It is indicated as an adjunct for prevention of organ transplant rejection and in severe rheumatoid arthritis. It has long been used as a steroid sparing agent in a variety of clinical scenarios [1,45]. In the United States azathioprine was usually combined with prednisone and CsA. Azathioprine was regarded as an adjunctive agent to CsA and the combination was often called "triple therapy". The term "adjunctive agent" is used to describe the immunosuppressive drugs that are used, or were developed for use, in combination with a calcineurin inhibitor to enhance the potency of the immunosuppressive protocol, as measured by a decreased incidence of acute rejection episodes [46].

2.5.1. Mechanism of action

Azathioprine inhibits purine metabolism. Following exposure to nucleophiles such as glutathione, azathioprine is cleaved to 6-mercaptopurine, which in turn is converted to additional metabolites that inhibit *de novo* purine synthesis. 6-thio-IMP, a fraudulent nucleotide, is converted to 6-thio-GMP and finally to 6-thio-GTP, which is incorporated into DNA. Cell proliferation is thereby inhibited, impairing a variety of lymphocyte functions. Azathioprine appears to be a more potent immunosuppressive agent than 6-mercaptopurine, which may reflect differences in drug uptake or pharmacokinetic differences in the resulting metabolites [1,45].

2.5.2. Side effects

The major side effect of azathioprine is bone marrow suppression, including leukopenia (common), and thrombocytopenia (less common). Other important adverse effects include increased susceptibility to infections (especially varicella and herpes simplex viruses) and hepatotoxicity [1].

2.6. Anti-IL-2 receptor (Anti-CD25) antibodies

There are two anti–IL-2R preparations for use in clinical transplantation: daclizumab and basiliximab. These are used for prophylaxis of acute organ rejection in adult patients. Basiliximab is considered a chimeric antibody, because it consists of approximately 70% human and 30% murine proteins. This agent has low immunogenicity potential due to the incorporation of human protein sequences. Daclizumab consists of 90% human and 10% murine components. The effectiveness of daclizumab is comparable to that of basiliximab, with an adverse-effect profile comparable to that seen with placebo [1,46].

2.6.1. Mechanism of action

Basiliximab binds with high affinity to the alpha subunit of the IL-2 receptor, also known as CD25, where it acts as a receptor antagonist. The antagonistic effect on the IL-2 receptor prevents T-cell activation and subsequent proliferation without causing lysis or cell destruction. Daclizumab, like basiliximab, is a nondepleting monoclonal antibody that acts as an antagonist at the CD25 subunit of T cells and received marketing approval in 1997 for induction therapy in renal transplant recipients. In Phase III trials, the half-life of daclizumab was 20 days, resulting in saturation of the IL-2Rα on circulating lymphocytes for up to 120 days after transplantation. In these trials, daclizumab was used with maintenance immunosuppression regimens (CsA, azathioprine, and steroids; CsA and steroids). Subsequently, daclizumab was successfully used with a maintenance triple-therapy regimen—either with CsA or TRL, steroids, and MMF substituting for azathioprine. In the Phase III trials, the half-life of basiliximab was 7 days. In one randomized trial, basiliximab was safe and effective when used in a maintenance regimen consisting of CsA, MMF, and prednisone [1,47].

2.6.2. Side effects

No cytokine-release syndrome has been observed with these antibodies, but anaphylactic reactions can occur. Although lymphoproliferative disorders and opportunistic infections may occur, as with the depleting antilymphocyte agents, the incidence ascribed to anti-CD25 treatment appears remarkably low. No significant drug interactions with anti–IL-2-receptor antibodies have been described [46,47].

2.7. Alemtuzumab

The antibody alemtuzumab is a recombinant DNA-derived humanized monoclonal antibody that is directed against the cell surface glycoprotein CD52, which is expressed on the surface of normal and malignant B and T lymphocytes, NK cells, monocytes, macrophages, and tissues of the male reproductive system; thus, the drug causes extensive lympholysis by inducing apoptosis of targeted cells. It has achieved some use in renal transplantation because it produces prolonged T- and B-cell depletion and allows drug minimization [1,47].

2.7.1. Mechanism of action

Alemtuzumab antibody binds to CD52, it triggers an antibody-dependent lysis of these cells. The depletion of lymphocytes is so marked that it takes several months or up to one year postadministration for a patient's immune system to be fully reconstituted ([1,47].

2.7.2. Side effects

Alemtuzumab's mechanism of depletion is so profound that its adverse-effect profile occurs frequently and with a high level of severity. Adverse effects associated with alemtuzumab use include neutropenia (70%), thrombocytopenia (52%), anemia (47%), nausea (54%), vomiting (41%), diarrhea (22%), headache (24%), dysesthesias (15%), dizziness (12%), and autoimmune hemolytic anemia (<5%) [47].

2.8. Glucocorticoids

The introduction of glucocorticoids as immunosuppressive drugs in the 1960s played a key role in making organ transplantation possible. Steroids are a cornerstone of immunosuppressive therapy in kidney transplantation despite their side effects and morbidity. More than 95% of transplant recipients are treated with steroids as a usual component of clinical immunosuppressive regimens. Prednisone, prednisolone, and other glucocorticoids are used alone and in combination with other immunosuppressive agents for treatment of transplant rejection and autoimmune disorders [1,48]. Transplantation specialists are now moving toward protocols that reduce the incidence of infections and minimize adverse events. Most immunosuppressive regimens are currently based on the combination of calcineurin inhibitors (CsA, TRL) with antiproliferative agents (azathioprine, MMF) and steroids (prednisone) [49].

2.8.1. Mechanism of action

Glucocorticoids lyse (in some species) and induce the redistribution of lymphocytes, causing a rapid, transient decrease in peripheral blood lymphocyte counts. To effect longer-term responses, steroids bind to receptors inside cells; either these receptors, glucocorticoid-induced proteins, or interacting proteins regulate the transcription of numerous other genes. Additionally, glucocorticoid-receptor complexes increase IκB expression, thereby curtailing activation of NF-κB, which increases apoptosis of activated cells. Of central importance, key proinflammatory cytokines such as IL-1 and IL-6 are down regulated. T cells are inhibited from making IL-2 and proliferating. The activation of cytotoxic T lymphocytes is inhibited. Neutrophils and monocytes display poor chemotaxis and decreased lysosomal enzyme release. Therefore, glucocorticoids have broad anti-inflammatory effects on multiple components of cellular immunity [1].

2.8.2. Side effects

Steroids are effective in reducing the incidence of acute rejection but are an important cause of morbidity and probably mortality. Moreover, they have adverse effects on cardiovascular risk factors such as hypertension, hyperglycemia, or hyperlipidemia, deleterious effects on bone metabolism, and may contribute to an increased risk of infection [1,48].

3. General principles of Therapeutic Drug Monitoring (TDM)

A basic tenet of clinical pharmacology is that the pharmacologic activity of an exogenously administered agent is related to the free drug concentration available at its receptor or ligand-binding site. A mayor underlying hypothesis in clinical pharmacokinetics is that the concentration of the agent in blood, serum or some other measurable compartment is related to the concentration of free (or non-bound) drug at its effector site [50]. Drugs are administered to achieve a therapeutic objective. Once this objective is defined, a drug and its dosage regimen are chosen for the patient. Drug therapy is subsequently managed together with steps required to initiate therapy, this management is usually accomplished by monitoring incidence and intensity of both therapeutic and toxic effects.

3.1. Therapeutic range

The therapeutic range (therapeutic index) is the ratio between the toxic dose and the therapeutic dose of a drug. The closer this ratio is to 1, the more difficult the drug is to use in clinical practice. The therapeutic index for immunosuppressant drugs is very low, whereas that for amoxicillin is extremely high. Clinical use of drugs with a narrow therapeutic index has led to the monitoring of drug concentrations in patients – therapeutic drug monitoring – in which the plasma concentration of a drug is measured and the dose adjusted to achieve a desired therapeutic drug concentration. Generally defined as the range of drug concentrations associated with maximal efficacy and minimal toxicity, there is currently no standard defining an acceptable level of toxicity or efficacy, nor are there consistent procedures used to establish a therapeutic range [51].

In general, a therapeutic range should never be considered in absolute terms, as it represents no more than a combination of probability charts. In other words, a therapeutic range is a range of drug concentrations within which the probability of the desired clinical response is relatively high and the probability of unacceptable toxicity is relatively low [52].

Since the development of the range is probabilistic in nature, a concentration that is within the "therapeutic range" for a given drug does not exclude the possibility that signs and symptoms of toxicity experienced by an individual patient are related to the monitored drug. A concentration outside of the range also does not indicate that a patient will experience toxicity or reduced efficacy; however, the likelihood of either is certainly lower [51]. It is important to recognize that the therapeutic range is not necessarily valid outside of the population used to establish it. This is particularly critical for immunosuppressive drugs, as most patients that are treated with these drugs receive additional immunosuppressive agents. A change in dosing of one drug may have a profound impact on the pharmacodynamic relationship of another. The nature of the transplanted organ (e.g., cadaveric versus living-related donor kidneys), age, and co-morbid illness can all have important influences on the pharmacodynamic response. The importance of these factors should not be ignored [51].

3.2. Interpretation of plasma drug concentration

The process of selecting the most appropriate dosage regimen to achieve concentrations in a relatively narrow range may be complicated by unpredictable intrapatient and interpatient variability in the drug's pharmacokinetics. A sophisticated application of pharmacokinetic principles, incorporating prior and subsequent measures of drug concentration and effects, can improve the quality of one's predictions. Although a single "best" approach to using drug concentrations does not exist for every drug, it is imperative to realize that without a systematic approach to therapeutic drug concentration monitoring, drug concentrations may be uninterpretable, unhelpful and potentially harmful. It thus becomes essential to recognize the key elements of clinical pharmacokinetics and pharmacodynamics, and to develop strategies to perform and use them most effectively [52].

There are a number of advantages to therapeutic drug monitoring that provide the clinician with clinically useful information. Plasma drug concentrations in conjunction with a thorough assessment of the patient's clinical status and the therapeutic goals to be achieved provide a means of successfully and rapidly individualizing a patient's therapeutic regimen to assure optimal benefits con minimal risk. Therapeutic drug measuring is only one part of therapeutic drug monitoring that provides expert clinical interpretation of drug concentration as well as evaluation based on pharmacokinetic principles. Expert interpretation of a drug concentration measurement is essential to ensure full clinical benefit. Clinicians routinely monitor drug pharmacodynamics by directly measuring the physiological indices of therapeutic responses, such as lipid concentrations, blood glucose, blood pressure, and clotting [53].

Anyone involved in the utilization of information derived from TDM must always bear in mind that the interpretation of plasma drug concentration must always be carried out in conjunction with an assessment of the clinical status of the patient. Therapeutic ranges should more correctly be described as optimal concentrations. According to the definition mentioned above, the therapeutic range (optimal concentration) of a drug is that concentration of drug present in plasma or some other biologic fluid or tissue that provides the desired therapeutic response in most patients. The severity of the disease process determines the amount of drug necessary to achieve a given therapeutic effect. Thus, it is quite possible that a patient may achieve the desired therapeutic effect at a plasma concentration well below the optimal range. Conversely, some patients will not achieve the desired therapeutic effect even when plasma concentrations are elevated into the toxic range. If the desired therapeutic effect is achieved at suboptimal plasma concentrations, every attempt should be made to avoid the prescription of additional drugs simply to increase the plasma concentration into what is commonly referred to as the therapeutic range. Obviously, the interpretation of plasma drug concentration must take into account the various factors that can alter the steady state plasma concentrations achieved on a given dosage form [54].

3.3. Therapeutic Drug Monitoring (TDM)

Individualizing a patient's drug therapy to obtain the optimum balance between therapeutic efficacy and the occurrence of adverse events is the physician's goal. However, achieving this goal is not always straight forward, being complicated by within and between patient variability in both pharmacokinetics and pharmacodynamics. In the early 1960's new analytical techniques became available allowing the measurement of the low drug concentrations seen in biological fluids during drug treatment. This offered the opportunity to reduce the pharmacokinetic component of variability by controlling drug therapy using concentrations in the body rather than by dose alone. This process became known as therapeutic drug monitoring [55].

The aim of TDM is to optimize pharmacotherapy by maximizing therapeutic efficacy, while minimizing adverse events, in those instances where the blood concentration of the drug is a better predictor of the desired effect(s) than the dose. The reasons why these principles have gained wide acceptance include the following: (1) although imperfect, a better relationship often exists between the effect of a given drug and its concentration in the blood than between the dose of the drug and the effect; (2) a thorough understanding of pharmacokinetics, i.e., the processes of drug absorption, distribution, metabolism, and drug excretion in individual patients and in patient populations is available; and (3) the development of reliable and relatively easy to use drug-monitoring assays. In addition, TDM can also be useful in cases in which compliance is in question, where it is not clear if the right drug is being taken, where dosage adjustment is required as a result of drug–drug or drug–food interactions, and where intoxication is suspected.

TDM is more than simply the analysis of a single drug concentration in the blood of a patient and a report of this number. It also comprises interpretation of the value measured using the mathematical (pharmacokinetic) principles mentioned above, drawing the appropriate conclusions about the result, and advising the physician who ordered the test how to optimize treatment. It is important to apply a uniform definition of TDM here, because different definitions have previously been used in cost-effectiveness studies and reviews of TDM. Consequently, comparisons have been made based on different approaches, which may influence the results. The International Association for Therapeutic Drug Monitoring and Clinical Toxicology has adopted the following definition:

Therapeutic drug monitoring is defined as the measurement made in the laboratory of a parameter that, with appropriate interpretation, will directly influence prescribing procedures. Commonly the measurement is in a biologic matrix of a prescribed xenobiotic, but it may also be of an endogenous compound prescribed as replacement therapy in an individual who is physiologically or pathologically deficient in that compound. This definition places TDM within the total therapeutic approach and should give not only more emphasis to the medication and patient-safety aspects of pharmacotherapy, but also more insight into why there are differences in efficacy among different patients. This definition implies that clinical pharmacologists have an active involvement in drug therapy, something that is not yet realized in many countries [56].

3.3.1. Why TDM for immunosuppressants?

For a drug to be a suitable candidate for therapeutic drug monitoring it must satisfy the following criteria [55]:

1. There should be a clear relationship between drug concentration and effect.

2. The drug should have a narrow therapeutic index; that is, the difference in the concentrations exerting therapeutic benefit and dose causing adverse events should be small.

3. There should be considerable between-subject pharmacokinetic variability and, therefore, a poor relationship between dose and drug concentration/response.

4. The pharmacological response of the drug should be difficult to assess or to distinguish form adverse events.

The most commonly used immunosuppressants require TDM because of their narrow therapeutic index and significant variability in blood concentrations between individuals. In transplant recipients, both supratherapeutics and subtherapeutics drug concentrations can have devastating results. At subtherapeutics drug concentrations, the transplant recipient is at risk for allograft rejection. At supratherapeutics drug concentrations, the patient is at risk for over-immunosuppression which can potentially lead to infection or drug specific side effects. It is it known that neurological and gastrointestinal side effects occur more frequently at higher concentrations of TRL [53]. Immunosuppressants display significant interindividual variability in plasma drug concentrations, which creates the demand for TDM when such drugs are used.

3.3.2. Factors contributing to the variability

Immunosuppressants display significant interindividual variability in plasma drug concentrations, which creates the demand for TDM when such drugs are used. It is appropriate to look into the multitude of factors that contribute to the interindividual variability. Some of the factors include drug-nutrients interactions, drug-disease interactions, renal insufficiency, inflammation and infection, gender, age, polymorphism and liver mass. Drug nutrient interactions are becoming very widely appreciated. The metabolism of drugs sometimes also depends on the type of diet taken by the patients. Renal transplant patients may have reduced oral bioavailability for TRL. When given with meals, especially with high fat content food, oral bioavailability of TRL decreases [57].

To avoid the possible effect of food on TRL bioavailability, the drug should be given at a constant time in relation to meals. Several studies have demonstrated that grapefruit juice can increase plasma concentrations of CsA by inhibiting CYP3A-mediated metabolism and by increasing drug absorption via inhibition of P-glycoprotein (P-gp) efflux transporters. Also, oral TRL should not be taken with grapefruit juice since this vehicle inhibits CYP3A4 and/or P-gp contained in the gastrointestinal tract and markedly increases bioavailability. Similarly, drug disease interactions can also contribute to interindividual variability in plasma concentration of immunosuppressants. Renal insufficiency can result in an altered free fraction of MPA due to the reduction in protein binding. MMF is rapidly converted to its active form, MPA, upon reaching the systemic circulation. MPA is metabolized to its glucuronide metabolite, MPA glucuronide (MPAG), by glucoronyl transferases in the liver and possibly elsewhere. MPAG is then excreted by the kidney. MPA is extensively and avidly bound to serum albumin. Previous studies have demonstrated that it is only the free (non-protein-bound) fraction of MPA that is available to exert its action. *In vivo* and *in vitro* studies demonstrate that renal insufficiency decreases the protein binding of MPA and increases free drug concentrations. This decrease in protein binding seems to be caused both by the uremic state itself and by competition with the retained metabolite MPAG. The disposition of MPA in patients with severe renal impairment may be significantly affected by this change in protein binding [58]. The concomitant administration of TRL and nonsteroidal anti-inflammatory drugs has been described as a possible cause of increased TRL nephrotoxicity because of the reduction of vasodilator prostaglandin synthesis through a blockade of the enzyme cyclo-oxygenase. Coadministration of ibuprofen and TRL has resulted in acute renal failure. Drugs such as aminoglycosides, cotrimoxazole (trimethoprim/sulfamethoxazole), amphotericin B and aciclovir, which cause significant renal dysfunction on their own, may also enhance TRL nephrotoxicity in the absence of careful monitoring of both renal function and drug concentrations [59].

It has been demonstrated that the *in vitro* metabolism of CsA in human liver microsomes was significantly reduced by TRL [60]. Interaction between MMF and TRL or CsA is probably related to a possible inhibitory effect of TRL on MPA metabolism and an inhibition of the enterohepatic recirculation of MPA by CsA, resulting in a substantial reduction in the MMF dosage when associated with TRL as compared with CsA. This has been reported in pediatric renal allograft patients and animal models [61,62].

Gender also influences drug concentration. Biologic differences exist between men and women that can result in differences in responses to drugs. Both pharmacokinetic and pharmacodynamic differences between the sexes exist, with more data on pharmacokinetic differences. Bioavailability after oral drug dosing, for CYP3A substrates in particular, may be somewhat higher in women compared to men [63]. It is known that MPA is primarily metabolized in the liver to its MPAG derivative. Morissette et al., found that men treated with MMF and TRL showed a lower ratio than patients treated with this couple of drugs, confirming that TRL inhibits glucuronidation of MPA. Because MPAG can favor the elimination of MPA, they concluded that gender differences and cotreatment with TRL must be taken into consideration when MMF is being administered [64]. Velickovic et al., investigated the gender differences in pharmacokinetics of TRL, their result show remarkable gender-related differences between women and men after the first oral dose among kidney transplant recipients on quaternary immunosuppressive therapy, including TRL, MMF, methylprednisolone and basiliximab [65].

Likewise, age can also contribute to interindividual difference in immunosuppressant plasma concentration. Pharmacokinetic parameters observed in adults may not be applicable to children, especially to the younger age groups. In general, patients younger than 5 years of age show higher clearance rates regardless of the organ transplanted or the immunosuppressive drug used [66]. Young children (1–6 years of age) appear to need higher doses per kilogram body weight of TRL than older children and adults to maintain similar trough concentrations. The reason for this age-related faster clearance rate is unknown [67]. Pediatric transplant recipients require higher doses of CsA to maintain blood concentrations equal to those found in adults [68]. Studies using intravenous CsA demonstrate that this is not because of any metabolic differences, as CsA clearance is not related to age [69].

Polymorphism has demonstrated functional consequences of many drug metabolizing enzymes. For example, CsA is known substrate for CYP3A4/5 and P-gp. CYP3A5 is one of the main CYP3A enzymes and its expression is clearly polymorphic and shows ethnic dependence. TRL is primarily metabolized by cytochrome P450(CYP)3A enzymes in the gut wall and liver. It is also a substrate for P-gp, which counter-transports diffused TRL out of intestinal cells and back into the gut lumen. Age-associated alterations in CYP3A and P-gp expression and/or activity, along with liver mass and body composition changes would be expected to affect the pharmacokinetics of TRL in the elderly [70]. The importance of interethnic differences in the pharmacokinetics of immunosuppressants has been recognized as having a significant impact on the outcome of transplantation. In a retrospective analysis Fitzimmons et al., found that the oral bioavailability of TRL in African American healthy volunteers and kidney transplant patients was significantly lower than in non-African Americans, but there was no statistically significant difference in clearance [71]. These results were confirmed in a healthy volunteer study. The absolute oral bioavailability of TRL in African American and Latin American subjects was significantly lower than in Caucasians. The results suggested that the observed ethnic differences in TRL pharmacokinetics were, instead, related to differences in intestinal P-glycoprotein-mediated efflux and CYP3A-mediated metabolism rather than differences in hepatic elimination [72].

Other ethnic groups such as the Japanese populations are not different from the Caucasian population because their transplant outcomes were comparable under usual TRL dosages [73]. All this factors contribute to the variability of immunosuppressant concentrations which has to be maintained within therapeutic range in order to achieve the optimal benefit of drug therapy, rendering TDM necessary for these drugs.

4. Monitoring of individual immunosuppressive agents

4.1. Cyclosporine (CsA)

The introduction of CsA in the early 1980s was immediately associated with an enhanced one year renal allograft survival; however, the argument for the therapeutic monitoring to optimize efficacy and safety, has been discussed in the last 25 years and it is still debated [74].

4.1.1. Therapeutic monitoring

4.1.1.1. Trough concentration (C_0) monitoring

Over the past two decades, there have been changes to recommended CsA dosing, changes in concomitant medications, and one major change to the oral drug formulation. Lately, there has also been the introduction of generic formulations of CsA [75]. In 1988, in a prospective study showed that although C_0 (trough concentration) levels of CsA correlated poorly with dose, Cmax was significantly correlated with dose, Area Under the Curve (AUC) and elimination half-life ($t_{1/2}$). Those who suffered acute rejection had a significantly lower Cmax by 15–31% [76]. The problem with this method for adjusting the dosage of CsA is that it relies on only one aspect of CsA pharmacokinetics, the predose or trough concentration. With the original formulation of CsA, Sandimmune®, this was the best practice, but during the conversion of patients from that formulation to the improved formulation, Neoral® the 2 h post-dose concentration has been advocated as a single concentration monitoring alternative to C0 [77]. The microemulsion formulation of CsA, Neoral®, makes CsA pharmacokinetics more predictable and reduces the effects of bile and food on absorption [78]. Nevertheless the predose concentration is still widely used in clinical practice. Currently, most transplant centers measure a single steady-state CsA concentration as either a C_0 predose trough or 2 hours postdose, while some conduct multiple measurements to determine CsA AUC estimates [79]. The target predose concentrations varied not only with transplanted organ and time after transplant but also with the analytical method used. The therapeutic range of CsA used by clinicians varies greatly according to the type of assay used to measure CsA and whether blood or serum concentrations are determined by the clinical laboratory.

Thus, it has reported by high pressure liquid chromatography, monoclonal fluorescence polarization immunoassay (monoclonal TDx assay, Abbott Diagnostics®), or monoclonal radioimmunoassay (various manufacturers), the level of therapeutic concentrations in blood are 10-400 ng/mL. By high pressure liquid chromatography, monoclonal fluorescence polarization immunoassay (monoclonal TDx assay, Abbott Diagnostics®), or monoclonal radioimmunoassay (various manufacturers), the level of therapeutic concentrations in serum are 50-150 ng/mL. By polyclonal fluorescence polarization immunoassay (monoclonal TDx assay, Abbott Diagnostics®), or polyclonal radioimmunoassay (various manufacturers) the level of therapeutic concentrations in blood are 200-800 ng/mL, and by polyclonal fluorescence polarization immunoassay (monoclonal TDx assay, Abbott Diagnostics®), or polyclonal radioimmunoassay (various manufacturers), the level of therapeutic concentrations in plasma are 100-400 ng/mL [79].

4.1.1.2. Area under the blood concentration-time curve (AUC)

The first steps towards the development of a more precise monitoring strategy for CsA resulted from the landmark studies by Lindholm and Kahan and Kahan et al., which identified a link between the pharmacokinetics of CsA and clinical outcomes in the individual transplant recipient [80,81]. The area under the concentration-time curve for CsA over a 12-hour drug administration interval (AUC_{0-12h}) was a more precise predictor of graft loss and incidence of acute rejection than other parameters, including the C_0. Since then, subsequent studies on the pharmacokinetics of CsA in renal transplant patients have identified that intrapatient variability in AUC values over time was directly correlated with the risk of chronic rejection [77,82].

Proper calculation of AUC requires administration of a dose, followed by blood collection according to an intensive sampling strategy. Concentration values obtained are used to calculate AUC, usually by the trapezoidal method [78]. Some advantages of AUC monitoring are that it is the most precise indicator of drug exposure, can characterize abnormal absorption patterns, appears to be a predictor of clinical outcomes, generates a concentration-time profile, allows calculation of oral pharmacokinetic parameters, and reduces the problems associated with laboratory errors and single concentrations [74,83,84].

Despite its appealing potential advantages, the major disadvantage of AUC monitoring is its inherent need for multiple blood samples. The increased number of samples required, makes AUC monitoring impractical for routine clinical use, more expensive in the short term because of increased sample collection, analysis and interpretation of results, and inconvenient for patients, especially those in an outpatient setting [77,85]. AUC has been advocated as a better parameter to monitor than trough concentrations, because trough concentrations give no indication of exposure to CsA. For example, 2 patients could have the same trough concentration, but one could have a much lower AUC and, therefore, exposure to CsA. Unfortunately, AUC monitoring is not clinically feasible because of the added time, expense and inconvenience required to collect a sufficient number of samples to properly calculate AUC. Although the full AUC for CsA has been demonstrated as being a sensitive monitoring tool, there may be an alternative approach to the determination of the degree and variability of CsA exposure in the individual patient [77,83].

4.1.1.3. Two hours post dose concentration monitoring (C_2)

This approach, which is termed 'absorption profiling', has the underlying rationale that the 4-hour absorption phase following administration provides measurements that are more informative than C_0 monitoring in the assessment of likely CsA exposure and subsequent clinical response [86,87]. AUC_{0-4h} monitoring is a sensitive tool used to optimize CsA immunosuppression in renal transplant recipients. However, the tool is not practical in the clinical setting because of 3 drawbacks: (1) it requires multiple sampling of blood for determination of the AUC_{0-4h}, (2) the actual value requires a mathematical calculation step, and (3) the test may be too expensive for many clinical hospitals or institutions because of the use of added costly laboratory tests for CsA concentrations and the subsequent increase in workload. Therefore, the search for a single blood-sampling point that best reflects the sensitivity of AUC_{0-4h} was the focus of several research initiatives that resulted in a broad approval for C_2 monitoring [82,85]. This method is done by measuring either the area under the blood CsA concentration-time curve in the first hours after dose, AUC_{0-4} or, more simply, by measuring the blood CsA concentration at 2 hours after dose, C_2 [82].

In *the novo* patients this monitoring method has led to result in the following clinical benefits compared with trough concentration monitoring [88]: (1) reduced incidence of acute rejection, (2) reduced severity of rejection episodes and (3) reduced incidence of nephrotoxicity.

4.1.1.4. Bayesian forecasting

The initial pharmacokinetic models for CsA were complicated by the nonlinear, segmented, zero order absorption of the drug from the gut [77,89]. Bayesian forecasting is a TDM tool that has been successfully used clinically in the monitoring of drugs that have a narrow therapeutic index, including antiepileptic drugs, theophylline and aminoglycosides; however, although Bayesian forecasting has proven useful clinically with other drugs, this is not the case with CsA [78]. Bayesian forecasting, in its modern form, was first proposed in 1979 by Sheiner et al. [90]. Since that time, user-friendly computer programs that perform this technique have become widely available. These programs are capable of calculating dosage regimens and pharmacokinetic parameters, as well as predicting drug concentrations by blending population values with patient-specific values [78]. However, these methods were technically complex and were not practical or successful for individualizing CsA therapy in a routine clinical setting and therefore did not gain widespread use. The introduction of Neoral, with its less variable and more predictable blood concentration profile, has rekindled interest in the pharmacokinetic modeling of CsA and in the use of Bayesian forecasting to predict CsA blood concentrations [77].

4.2. Tacrolimus (TRL)

The therapeutic range for TRL used by most transplantation centers is 5–20 ng/mL in blood. Although, plasma TRL concentrations have been measured and an equivalent therapeutic range in this matrix suggested (0.5–2 ng/mL), the two most widely used assays for the drug use blood samples. Because this drug is extensively bound to erythrocytes, blood concentrations average about 15 times greater than concurrently measured serum or plasma concentrations [57,79,91]. As a result, whole blood has become the principal sample used for TRL concentration monitoring, with extraction accomplished through cell lysis and protein denaturation steps that are similar or identical to those used for CsA analysis [51]. The pharmacokinetics of TRL is highly variable. Since TRL shares many of the pharmacokinetic and pharmacodynamic problems associated with CsA the rationale for TDM is similar. Although the feasibility of a limited sampling scheme to predict AUC has been demonstrated, as yet, through or predose whole blood concentration monitoring is still the method of choice [55].

4.2.1. Therapeutic monitoring

TRL whole-blood through concentrations have been found to correlate well with the area under the concentration-time curve measurements in liver, kidney and bone marrow transplant recipients (r= 0.91-0.99). Thus, through concentrations are good index of overall drug exposure, and are currently used for routine monitoring as part of patient care posttransplantation [91,92]. This approach offers the opportunity to reduce the pharmacokinetic variability by implementing drug dose adjustments based on plasma/blood concentrations. Drug levels are obtained as predose (12 hours after previous dose) trough concentrations in whole blood [88]. These trough levels correlate reasonably well with area under the curve, with total area under the curve being an accurate measure of drug exposure [94].

Therapeutic ranges of TRL after kidney transplantation are reported as a range for various times after transplant: 0-1 month, 15-20 μg/L; 1-3 months, 10-15 μg/L; and more than 3 months, 5-12 μg/L [95]. TRL blood concentrations are monitored 3 to 7 days a week for the first 2 weeks, at least three times for the following 2 weeks, and whenever the patient comes for an outpatient visit thereafter [96]. On the basis of the terminal half-life of TRL, it was suggested to start monitoring blood concentrations 2 to 3 days after initiation of TRL treatment after the drug has reached steady state. However it is important to reach effective drug concentrations early after transplantation to decrease the risk of acute rejection and to avoid excessive early calcineurin inhibitors concentrations that may be severely damaging after reperfusion of the transplanted organ [97].

The frequency of TDM of TRL should be increased in the case of suspected adverse events or rejection, when liver function is deteriorating, after dose adjustments of the immunosuppressants, change of route of administration, or change of drug formulations, when drugs that are known to interact with CYP3A or P-gP are added or discontinued, or when their doses are changed, in case of severe illness that may affect drug absorption or elimination such as severe immune reactions and sepsis, or if noncompliance is suspected [98].

4.3. Mycophenolic acid (MPA)

In 1995, for preventing rejection in renal transplant patients, MMF, the morpholinoethyl ester prodrug from MPA was approved for clinical use. This drug has since become the predominant anti-metabolite immunosuppressive used in the transplant setting. Although the current labeling information for MMF does not indicate any need for therapeutic monitoring of plasma MPA concentrations, there were a number of studies showing a relationship between MPA pharmacokinetics and clinical outcome [99]. Definitive determination of the pharmacokinetics of the drug in renal allograft recipients after transplantation is not without difficulty. In principle, substantial changes in pharmacokinetics could be produced by changes following transplantation, both in the immediate post-transplant period (reflecting rapid alterations in drug therapy, renal function, hemodynamics and gastrointestinal motility) as well as more gradual changes (reflecting change in bodyweight, plasma proteins and organ function) [100]. The greatest variability in MPA pharmacokinetic is noted in the initial 2 months following transplantation, when adequate immunosuppression is critical to graft function and survival. It has also become apparent from longer term pharmacokinetic studies that exposure to MPA increases over time due to reduced clearance of the drug. A possible additional factor that could con-tribute to the higher oral clearance of MPA early after transplantation is corticosteroid therapy, which is significantly higher in that period but then is tapered to low dose lev-els or completely withdrawn. Based upon the marked pharmacokinetic variability ob-served with MPA and the pharmacodynamic relationship of pharmacokinetic parameters to rejection outcome, several scientific societies and consensus conferences have advocat-ed the use of concentration monitoring for patients undergoing treatment with MMF or enteric-coated MPA [101].

4.3.1. Therapeutic monitoring

The incorporation of MMF into immunosuppressive regimens has been associated with decrease rates of acute rejection and decreased chronic allograft loss. Indications for TDM of mycophenolates were reviewed in a consensus meeting [101]. They included high-risk patients, patients with delayed graft function, or patients with immunosuppressive protocols excluding induction therapy or steroids or calcineurin inhibitor or patients with calcineurin minimization. Most of these patients (especially high-risk patients) are often excluded from the clinical trials. In fact, MPA TDM is currently only used in a few transplant centers on a routine basis, whereas a few others only checked MPA exposure in case of unexpected acute rejection or adverse event or drug interaction. Most of the centers never measure MPA. It is clear that the use of MPA TDM is conditioned by the faith of the physicians in its use, local availability of MPA measurements, and organization of the nursing staff [102].

4.3.1.1. Trough concentration (C$_0$) monitoring

Although a relationship between AUC and outcome exists, the clinical utility of concentration monitoring, particularly C$_0$ monitoring for MMF, has been questioned. Over the past decade, several studies were conducted to evaluate the clinical utility of prospective concentration controlled MMF therapy. While these studies were anticipated to fully clarify the utility of monitored MMF therapy, the outcomes from these studies are conflicting and have done little to settle the controversies surrounding this area of therapeutic drug monitoring [100]. With trough concentration, plasma concentration of MPA is measured immediately before a dose, it is easy to measure because only -ask patient to return to give sample, it is immediately before a dose, and only requires single simple possible association between C$_0$ and decreased rejection noted in transplant recipients. However this method represents some disadvantages. Timing may not be accurate (depends on remembering time of last dose). Timing may vary from the "ideal" (12 h after last dose) by several hours. There is no high-level evidence of a strong association between C$_0$ and outcome, or between C$_0$ and AUC$_{0-12}$, C$_0$ is not a very informative time point for estimation of individual pharmacokinetic parameters. Single time-point samples such as the trough concentration or others do not correlate well with the MPA AUC, especially in the early posttransplantation period [103].

4.3.1.2. Limited sampling strategies for estimation of MPA AUC

The dose interval MPA AUC_{0-12} h is generally regarded as the most reliable pharmacokinetic parameter index of risk for acute rejection but is impractical to measure in routine clinical practice. Single time-point samples such as the trough concentration or others, do not correlate well with the MPA AUC, especially in the early posttransplantation period renal transplant patients and for regimens that include MMF plus CsA, TRL, or SRL [104]. Therefore, assessment of whether C_0 concentrations or other single time points correlate well with the AUC is important for establishing routine monitoring of the drug. Apart of the C_0 level other single time points after MMF dosing are examined for their ability to predict full AUC values. A full MPA AUC typically requires at least eight blood samples during 12 hour dose interval. In clinical practice this is impractical; therefore, abbreviated sampling schemes involving the collection of there to five plasma samples have been investigated. The abbreviated sampling approach has provided estimations of MPA AUC with high correlations ($r^2>0.8$). Several models have been developed all of them in renal transplant patients [105-108].

4.4. Sirolimus (SRL)

SRL (formerly known as rapamycin) is a macrolide antibiotic with immunosuppressive properties that was introduced relatively recently (September 1999) into clinical practice for maintenance therapy in organ transplantation [109]. Pharmacokinetics studies of SRL in renal transplant patients have been shown great variability between patients. Several features contribute to the interpatient pharmacokinetic variability observed with SRL and can include any combination of the following: absorption, distribution, metabolism and/or excretion [110].

This drug presents a rapid gastrointestinal absorption (t_{max} from 0.33 to 5 hours) as well as a low (mean value 14%) and variable bioavailability. It has been reported that SRL is a substrate for the multidrug P-glycoprotein transporter and that the biotransformation of SRL is mediated by CYP3A enzymes. Accordingly, considerable variability in its pharmacokinetic parameters may be expected (apparent blood clearance rates after oral administration from 87 to 416 mL/h/kg). In addition, the disposition of SRL in humans includes a large volume of distribution, a long half-life (35 to 95 hours) and dose proportionality for Cmax and AUC. Also, some interracial variability and an influence of hepatic dysfunction have been noted with SRL [111]. Although structurally similar to TRL, SRL has a novel mechanism of action, which leads to synergy with CsA. The long half-life of the drug necessitates a loading dose to achieve therapeutic concentrations quickly, and also allows for once daily administration. Highly variable absorption and metabolism of the drug result in large differences in blood concentrations among patients receiving the same dose. Efficacy for the prevention of acute rejection episodes, and the rate of common adverse effects (thrombocytopenia, leucopenia and hypertriglyceridemia), are concentration-dependent [112].

4.4.1. Therapeutic monitoring

Clinical data suggest that the immunosuppressive efficacy and the occurrence and severity of adverse effects of SRL correlate with blood concentrations [112]. Drug interactions with concomitant immunosuppressant medications will alter SRL whole blood concentrations. The appropriate SRL through concentration at steady state (Cmin,ss) for acute rejection episode prophylaxis is a function of the concomitant immunosuppressive regimen. When it is used as base therapy with azathioprine and prednisone, a regimen stipulating initial Cmin,ss values equal to 30 µg/L during the first 2 months, and 15 µg/L(LC/UV assay) thereafter, led to a 41% rate of acute rejection episodes among 41 cadaveric kidney transplant recipients [113].

When combined with MMF and prednisone, this SRL regimen was associated with a 27.5% rate of acute rejection episodes among 40 cadaveric renal transplant recipients. Indeed, the combination of SRL (Cmin,ss of 10 to 20 µg/L; LC/UV assay) and basiliximab with late introduction of low dosage CsA has provided excellent prophylaxis of acute rejection episodes and renal function for primary, non-African-American recipients of cadaveric kidney transplants that displayed delayed graft function [112,114,115].

In purely Caucasian low-risk liver and kidney-pancreas transplant recipients, Cmin,ss of 6 to 12 µg/L (IMx® assay) in combination with low dosage TRL has been reported to yield low rates of acute rejection episodes and toxicity [116]. Because of the long half-life and extensive tissue distribution of the drug, steady-state concentrations are not reached before day 6 after initiation of therapy or after a dosage change. Thus, daily concentration monitoring is not necessary; the first SRL measurements should not be obtained before day 4 after inception of, or change in therapy. Thereafter, recommend monitoring Cmin,ss weekly for the first month and bi-weekly for the next month, targeting a 5 to 15 µg/L range if CsA is being used concomitantly at Cmin,ss concentrations of 75 to 150 µg/L. If the patient fails to attain these values despite a dosage of 20mg/day, a full pharmacokinetic study should be performed to assess whether the defect is due to limited absorption or rapid clearance rates [112]. Modest correlation ($r = 0.59$) exists between SRL dose and peak plasma concentration (Cmax) or AUC, but a good correlation ($r = 0.85$) exists between trough concentration prior to the dose (minimum Cmin,ss and AUC. For this reason, Cmin,ss is a simple and useful index for therapeutic monitoring of SRL [112,117,118].

4.5. Everolimus (EVL)

In April 2010, EVL, a more water-soluble analog of SRL was approved for use in CsA-sparing regimens, including the requirement for adjusting EVL doses using target trough blood concentrations in renal transplant patients [51]. EVL, which has greater polarity than SRL, was developed in an attempt to improve the pharmacokinetic characteristics of SRL, particularly to increase its oral bioavailability. After a single oral dose of EVL 4mg in 12 healthy volunteers, it was absorbed rapidly (within 30 minutes after drug intake). The Cmax of EVL amounted to 44.2 ± 13.3 µg/L and was reached (t_{max}) after 30 minutes (range 0.5–1 hour). The AUC was 219 ± 69 µg* h/L. The overall absorption of EVL, like that of SRL, is probably affected by the activity of P-gp. It is recommended that patients should take the drug consistently with or without food to reduce fluctuations in drug exposure [119]. In an international study, the pharmacokinetics of EVL, were characterized over the first 6 months post-transplant in 731 patients receiving either 0.75 or 1.5mg bid EVL in addition to CsA and corticosteroids. The within- and between-patient variability of dose interval AUC was 27% and 31% respectively. There was no detectable influence of sex, age (16–66 years), or weight (42-132 kg) on AUC, but EVL exposure was significantly lower by an average of 20 % in blacks. In a study of 659 AUC profiles the correlation between trough concentration and overall exposure (AUC) there was a significant linear correlation with a regression coefficient of 0.89 and corresponding coefficient of determination of 0.79 [120].

For example, see [121] reported that multiple daily dosing of EVL, in doses up to 5 mg/day, is adequately well tolerated as add-on therapy in stable renal transplant patients receiving maintenance Neoral® immunosuppression. Similar degrees of correlation between EVL trough concentration and thrombocytopenia, leukopenia, hypertriglyceridemia, or hypercholesterolemia in 54 stable renal transplant patients (18-68 years) were found.

4.5.1. Therapeutic drug monitoring

EVL is a drug with a narrow therapeutic index. The limited and variable bioavailability, intrinsic interindividual pharmacokinetic variability, the number of factors affecting the pharmacokinetics, and the number of drug interactions limits the use of fixed doses of this drug. The EVL Cmin is a good surrogate marker of EVL exposure (AUC), and correlates with pharmacological response and clinical outcomes. Therefore, prospective dose adjustments to obtain and maintain a therapeutic EVL Cmin have the potential to improve efficacy and reduce toxicity [122].

A role for EVL drug monitoring has been suggested because of the potential for improving efficacy and reducing adverse effects, the EVL Cmin is a good surrogate marker of EVL exposure (AUC), and correlates with pharmacological response and clinical outcomes. Therefore, prospective dose adjustments to obtain and maintain a therapeutic EVL Cmin have the potential to improve efficacy and reduce toxicity [123]. Mere clinical monitoring of efficacy is insufficient because clinical presentations of graft rejection vary for each patient and are nonspecific. Thus, some authors have used a previously published 9-step decision-making algorithm to evaluate the utility of TDM for EVL. The recommended therapeutic range for EVL is a trough concentration of 3 to 8 ng/mL, as concentrations over 3 ng/mL have been associated with a decreased incidence of rejection, and concentrations >8 ng/mL with increased toxicity. Patients on EVL who have problems with absorption, who take concurrent cytochrome P450 inhibitors or inducers, or are noncompliant will attain the greatest benefit from therapeutic drug monitoring [124].

5. Advances in immunosuppression – Future trends

Maintenance immunosuppressive therapy over the past decade has become more diversified. Until the mid-1990s, CsA and azathioprine were the cornerstones in maintenance immunosuppressive therapy. Today, these agents have been largely replaced by the newer agents TRL and MMF. Triple immunosuppression continues to be the standard, and corticosteroids are still part of most widely used immunosuppressive protocols. More effective immunosuppression has reduced the incidence of acute rejection without a reduction in patient survival [125]. Calcineurin inhibitors are still the cornerstone of current immunosuppressive therapy, but have important cardiovascular and oncogenic side effects and nephrotoxicity effects that contributes to the multifactorial process called "chronic allograft dysfunction", the leading cause of chronic allograft failure among kidney transplant recipients. New drugs, with a different mechanism of action, are being developed focusing on a better balance between drug efficacy and toxicity. These novel compounds interfere with either T-cell mediated or antibody-mediated rejection [126].

A number of novel drugs are currently under investigation in Phase I, II, or III clinical trials primarily to replace the nephrotoxic but highly effective calcineurin inhibitors. ISA247 (voclosporine) is a CsA analog with reduced nephrotoxicity in Phase III study. AEB071 (sotrastaurin), a protein kinase C inhibitor, and CP-690550, a JAK3 inhibitor, are small molecules in Phase II studies EVL is derived from the mTOR inhibitor SRL and is in Phase III study. Belatacept is a humanized antibody that inhibits T-cell costimulation and has shown encouraging results in multiple Phase II and III trials. Alefacept and Efaluzimab are humanized antibodies that inhibit T-cell adhesion and are in Phase I and II clinical trials [127]. Finally, the exciting field of tissue engineering and stem cell biology with the repopulation of decellularized organs is ushering in a new paradigm for transplantation. The era of simplified immunosuppression regimens devoid of toxicities is upon us with the promise of dramatic improvement in long term survival [128].

6. Conclusions

Monitored drug therapy has undergone a tremendous change over the past quarter of a century with the increasing availability of advanced techniques like liquid chromatography with tandem mass spectrometry detection and immunoassays. Currently, the possibility of accurately and specifically measuring almost any drug in any biological fluid is a reality, and while TDM has become a standard of care for most immunosuppressive drugs, TDM practices will continue to evolve with the field of transplantation. New immunosuppressives, such as sotrastaurin, exhibit pharmacokinetic variability comparable to that seen with currently used immunosuppressive drugs and may benefit from monitoring therapy [129]. Although TDM of biologic drugs such as belatacept have not been reported in clinical trials to date, potentially useful pharmacodynamic assays that can be performed on blood specimens have been described [51,130]. The information gained through further study in these complex regimens should provide innovative strategies and new immunosuppressive agents that will serve to extend the functional life of allografts without toxicity or infection.

Author details

Ana Luisa Robles Piedras*, Minarda De la O Arciniega and Josefina Reynoso Vázquez

*Address all correspondence to: roblesa@uaeh.edu.mx

Academic Area of Pharmacy, Institute of Health Sciences, Autonomous University of Hidalgo State, Mexico

References

[1] Krensky AM, Vincenti F, Bennett WM. Immunosuppressants, Tolerogens, and Immunostimulants. In: Brunton L. (ed) Goodman and Gilman's The Pharmacological Basis of Therapeutics 11th ed. McGraw-Hill Co. New York, NY. 2006. p1405-1431.

[2] Kahan BD. Cyclosporine. New England Journal of Medicine 1989;32:1725-1738.

[3] Khanna A, Li B, Stenzel KH, Suthanthiran M. Regulation of new DNA synthesis in mammalian cells by cyclosporine. Demonstration of a transforming growth factor beta-dependent mechanism of inhibition of cell growth. Transplantation 1994;57:577-582.

[4] Freeman DJ. Pharmacology and pharmacokinetics of cyclosporine. Clinical Biochemistry 1991;24:9-14.

[5] Fairley JA. Intracellular targets of cyclosporine. Journal of the American Academy of Dermatology 1990;23:1329-1334.

[6] Halloran PF, Madrenas J. The mechanism of action of cyclosporine: a perspective for the 90's. Clinical Biochemistry 1991;24:3-7.

[7] Schreiber SL, Crabtree GR. The mechanism of action of cyclosporin A and FK506. Immunology Today 1992;13:136-142.

[8] Aszalos A. Cyclosporin: some aspects of its mode of action. A review. Journal of Medicine 1988;19:297-316.

[9] Product Information. Sandimmune® oral capsules, oral solution, intravenous injection, cyclosporine oral capsules, oral solution, intravenous injection. Novartis Pharmaceuticals Corporation, East Hanover, NJ. 2010.

[10] Cush JJ, Tugwell P, Weinblatt M, Yocum D. US consensus guidelines for the use of cyclosporin A in rheumatoid arthritis. Journal of Rheumatology 1999;26(5):1176-1186.

[11] Charnick SB, Nedelman JR, Chang CT, Hwang DS, Jin J, Moore MA, Wong R. Description of blood pressure changes in patients beginning cyclosporin A therapy. Therapeutic Drug Monitoring 1997;19:17-24.

[12] de Mattos AM, Olyaei AJ, Bennett WM. Nephrotoxicity of immunosuppressive drugs: long-term consequences and challenges for the future. American Journal of Kidney Diseases 2000;35(2):333-346.

[13] Ballantyne CM, Podet EJ, Patsch WP, Harati Y, Appel V, Gotto AM Jr, Young JB. Effects of cyclosporine therapy on plasma lipoprotein levels. The Journal of the American Medical Association 1989;262:53-56.

[14] McGaw WT, Porter H. Cyclosporine-induced gingival overgrowth: an ultrastructural stereologic study. Oral Surgery, Oral Medicine, Oral Pathology 1988;65(2):186-190.

[15] Daly CG. Resolution of cyclosporin A (CsA)-induced gingival enlargement following reduction in CsA dosage. Journal of Clinical Periodontology 1992;19:143-145.

[16] Wong W, Hodge MG, Lewis A, Sharpstone P, Kingswood JC. Resolution of cyclosporin-induced gingival hypertrophy with metronidazole. Lancet 1994;343:986.

[17] Shapiro R. Tacrolimus in pediatric renal transplantation: A review. Pediatric Transplantation 1998;2:270-276.

[18] Plosker GL. Foster RH. Tacrolimus: a further update of its pharmacology and therapeutic use in the management of organ transplantation. Drugs 2000;59:323-389.

[19] Tocci MJ, Matkovich DA, Collier KA, Kwok P, Dumont F, Lin S, Degudicibus S, Siekierka JJ, Chin J, Hutchinson NI. FK-506 selectively inhibits expression of early T cell activation genes. The Journal of Immunology 1989;143:718-726.

[20] Kay JE, Moore AL, Doe SE, Benzie CR, Schönbrunner R, Schmid FX, Halestrap AP. The mechanism of action of FK 506. Transplantation Proceedings 1990;22(1):96-99.

[21] Peters DH, Fitton A, Plosker GL, Faulds D. Tacrolimus: a review of its pharmacology, and therapeutic potential in hepatic and renal transplantation. Drugs 1993;46:746-794.

[22] Rauch MC, San Martín A, Ojeda D, Quezada C, Salas M, Cárcamo JG, Yañez AJ, Slebe JC, Claude A. Tacrolimus causes a blockage of protein secretion which reinforces its immunosuppressive activity and also explains some of its toxic side-effects. Tacrolimus causes a blockage of protein secretion which reinforces its immunosuppressive activity and also explains some of its toxic side-effects. Transplant Immunology 2009;22(1-2): 72-81.

[23] Product Information: PROGRAF® oral capsules, IV injection, tacrolimus oral capsules, IV injection. Astellas Pharma US, Inc. (per manufacturer), Deerfield, IL. 2011.

[24] Henry ML. Cyclosporine and tacrolimus (FK506): a comparison of efficacy and safety profiles. Clinical Transplantation 1999;13:209-220.

[25] Pham SM, Kormos RL, Hattler BG, Kawai A, Tsamandas AC, Demetris AJ, Murali S, Fricker FJ, Chang HC, Jain AB, Starzl TE, Hardesty RL, Griffith BP. A prospective trial of (FK 506) in clinical heart transplantation: intermediate-term results. The Journal of Thoracic and Cardiovascular Surgery 1996;111:764-772.

[26] AM, Furth SL, Case BW, Wise B, Colombani PM, Fivush BA. Evaluation of neurotoxicity in pediatric renal transplant recipients treated with tacrolimus (FK506). Clinical Transplantation 1997;11:412-414.

[27] Krentz AJ, Dousset B, Mayer D, McMaster P, Buckels J, Cramb R, Smith JM, Nattrass M. Metabolic effects of cyclosporin A and FK 506 in liver transplant recipients. Diabetes 1993;42:1753-1759.

[28] Ardestani F, Fatemi SS, Yakhchali B. Evaluation of mycophenolic acid production by Penicillium brevicompactum MUCL 19011 in batch and continuous submerged cultures. Biochemical Engineering Journal 2010;50(3):99-103.

[29] Oremus M, Zeidler J, Ensom MHH. Utility of monitoring mycophenolic acid in solid organ transplant patients. Evidence Report/Technology Assessment No. 164. AHRQ Publication No.08-E006. Rockville, MD: Agency for Healthcare Research and Quality. 2008.   http://www.ahrq.gov/downloads/pub/evidence/pdf/mpa/mpaorgan.pdf   (accessed 3 August 2012).

[30] Groth CG, Ohlman S, Gannedahl G, Ericzon BG. New immunosuppressive drugs in transplantation. Transplantation Proceedings 1993;25:2681-2683.

[31] Eugui EM, Mirkovich A, Allison AC. Lymphocyte-selective antiproliferative and immunosuppressive effects of mycophenolic acid in mice. Scandinavian Journal of Immunology 1991;33:175.

[32] Bumgardner GL, Roberts JP. New immunosuppressive agents. Gastroenterology Clinics of North America 1993;22:421-449.

[33] Butani L, Palmer J, Baluarte HJ, Polinsky MS. Adverse effects of mycophenolate mofetil in pediatric renal transplant recipients with presumed chronic rejection. Transplantation 1999;68:83-86.

[34] Product Information. CellCept® oral tablets, capsules, suspension and intravenous injection, mycophenolate mofetil oral tablets, capsules, suspension, mycophenolate mofetil hydrochloride intravenous injection. Roche Laboratories Inc., Nutley, NJ. 2009.

[35] Kuypers DR, Le Meur Y, Cantarovich M, Tredger MJ, Tett SE, Cattaneo D, Tönshoff B, Holt DW, Chapman J, Gelder T; Transplantation Society (TTS) Consensus Group on TDM of MPA. Consensus report on therapeutic drug monitoring of mycophenolic acid in solid organ transplantation. Clinical Journal of the American Society of Nephrology 2010;5:341-358.   http://ebookbrowse.com/transplante-consensus-report-therapeutic-drug-monitoring-mycophenolic-acid-pdf-d322644574 (accessed 3 August 2012).

[36] Watson CJ, Friend PJ, Jamieson NV, Frick TW, Alexander G, Gimson AE, Calne R. Sirolimus: a potent new immunosuppressant for liver transplantation. Transplantation 1999;67(4):505-509.   http://www.centerspan.org/pubs/transplantation/1999/0227/tr049900505o.pdf (accessed 3 August 2012).

[37] Kelly PA, Gruber SA, Behbod F, Kahan BD. Sirolimus, a new potent immunosuppressive agent. Pharmacotherapy 1997;17:1148-1156.

[38] Morris RE. Mechanisms of action of new immunosuppressive drugs. Kidney International 1996;49(53):S26-S38.

[39] Brattström C, Wilczek H, Tydén G, Böttiger Y, Säwe J, Groth CG. Hyperlipidemia in renal transplant recipients treated with sirolimus (Rapamycin). Transplantation 1998;65(9):1272-1274.

[40] Schuler W, Sedrani R, Cottens S, Häberlin B, Schulz M, Schuurman HJ, Zenke G, Zerwes HG, Schreier MH. SDZ RAD, a new rapamycin derivative. Transplantation 1997;64(1): 36-42.

[41] Eisen HJ, Tuzcu EM, Dorent R, Kobashigawa J, Mancini D, Valantine-von Kaeppler HA, Starling RC, Sørensen K, Hummel M, Lind JM, Abeywickrama KH, Bernhardt P; RAD B253 Study Group. RAD B253 Study Group. Everolimus for the prevention of allograft rejection and vasculopathy in cardiac-transplant recipients. The New England Journal of Medicine 2003;349:847-858.

[42] van Rossum HH, Romijn FP, Smit NP, de Fijter JW, van Pelt J. Everolimus and sirolimus antagonize tacrolimus based calcineurin inhibition via competition for FK-binding protein 12. Biochemical Pharmacology 2009;77(7):1206-1212.

[43] Sánchez-Fructuoso AI, Ruiz JC, Pérez-Flores I, Gómez Alamillo C, Calvo Romero N, Arias M. Comparative analysis of adverse events requiring suspension of mtor inhibitors: everolimus versus sirolimus. Transplantation Proceedings 2010;42(8): 3050-3052.

[44] Moldawer NP, Wood LS. Management of key adverse events associated with everolimus therapy. Kidney Cancer Journal 2010;8(2):51-59. http://www.kidney-cancer-journal.com/emag/v8n2/pageflip.htm (accessed 3 August 2012).

[45] Afzali B, Taylor AL, Goldsmith DJ. What we CAN do about chronic allograft nephropathy: Role of immunosuppressive modulations. Kidney International, 2005;68:2429-2443.

[46] Danovitch GM. Immunosuppressive medications for renal transplantation: A multiple choice question. Kidney International 2001; 59:388-402.

[47] Gabardi S, Martin ST, Roberts KL, Grafals M. Induction immunosuppressive therapies in renal transplantation. American Journal of Health-System Pharmacy 2011;68(1): 211-218.

[48] Helal I, Chan L. Steroid and calcineurin inhibitor-sparing protocols in kidney transplantation. Transplantation Proceedings 2011;43:472-477.

[49] Ponticelli C. Present and future of immunosuppressive therapy in kidney transplantation. Transplantation Proceedings 2011;43: 2439-2440.

[50] Budde K, Glander P. Pharmacokinetic principles of immunosuppressive drugs. Annals of Transplantation 2008;13(3):5-10.

[51] Milone MC., Shaw LMJ. Therapeutic Drug Monitoring for Immunosuppressive Agents. In: Kaplan B., Burkhart JG., Lakkis FG. (ed.) Immunotherapy in Transplantation: Principles and Practice. USA: Wiley-Blackwell; 2012. p95-113.

[52] Evans W. General Principles of Clinical Pharmacokinetics. In: Burton ME., Shaw LM., Schentag JJ., Evans WE. (ed) Applied Pharmacokinetics and Pharmacodynamics. Principles of Therapeutic Drug Monitoring. USA: Williams and Wilkins; 2006. p3-7.

[53] Kang JS, Lee MH. Overview of Therapeutic Drug Monitoring. The Korean Journal of Internal Medicine 2009;24(1):1-10. http://www.ncbi.nlm.nih.gov/pmc/articles/ PMC2687654/pdf/kjim-24-1.pdf (accessed 6 July 2012).

[54] Peppinger C., Massoud N. Therapeutic Drug Monitoring. In: Benet L., Massoud N., Gambertoglio J. (ed.) Pharmacokinetic Basis for Drug Treatment. New York: Raven Press; 1985. p367-393.

[55] Johnston A, Holt DW. Therapeutic drug monitoring of immunosuppressant drugs. British Journal of Clinical Pharmacology 1999; 47(4): 339–350.

[56] Neef C, Touw DJ, Stolk LM. Therapeutic Drug Monitoring in Clinical Research. Pharmaceutical Medicine.2008;22(4):235-44. http://adisonline.com/pharmaceuticalme-dicine/Abstract/2008/22040/Therapeutic_Drug_Monitoring_in_Clinical_Research. 4.aspx (accessed 6 July 2012).

[57] Venkataramanan R, Swaminathan A, Prasad T, Jain A, Zuckerman S, Warty V, McMichael J, Lever J, Burckart G, Starzl T. Clinical pharmacokinetics of tacrolimus. Clinical Pharmacokinetics 1995;29(6):404-30.

[58] Meier-Kriesche HU, Shaw LM, Korecka M, Kaplan B. Pharmacokinetics of mycophe-nolic acid in renal insufficiency. Therapeutic Drug Monitoring 2000;22(1):27-30.

[59] Mignat C. Clinically significant drug interactions with new immunosuppressive agents. Drug Safety 1997;16:267-78

[60] Omar G, Shah IA, Thomson AW, Whiting PH, Burke MD. FK 506 inhibition of cyclo-sporine metabolism by human liver microsomes. Transplantation Proceedings 1991;23(1 Pt 2):934-5.

[61] Filler G, Lampe D, Mai I, Strehlau J, Ehrich JH. Dosing of MMF in combination with tacrolimus for steroid-resistant vascular rejection in pediatric renal allografts. Trans-plant International 1998;11 Suppl 1:S82-5.

[62] van Gelder T, Klupp J, Barten MJ, Christians U, Morris RE. Comparison of the effects of tacrolimus and cyclosporine on the pharmacokinetics of mycophenolic acid. Therapeutic Drug Monitoring 2001;23(2):119-28.

[63] Schwartz JB. The influence of sex on pharmacokinetics. Clinical Pharmacokinetics 2003;42(2):107-21.

[64] Morissette P, Albert C, Busque S, St-Louis G, Vinet B. In vivo higher glucuronidation of mycophenolic acid in male than in female recipients of a cadaveric kidney allograft

and under immunosuppressive therapy with mycophenolate mofetil. Therapeutic Drug Monitoring 2001;23(5):520-5.

[65] Velicković-Radovanović R, Mikov M, Paunović G, Djordjević V, Stojanović M, Cvetković T, Djordjević AC. Gender differences in pharmacokinetics of tacrolimus and their clinical significance in kidney transplant recipients. Gender Medicine 2011;8(1):23-31.

[66] del Mar Fernández De Gatta M, Santos-Buelga D, Domínguez-Gil A, García MJ. Immunosuppressive therapy for paediatric transplant patients: pharmacokinetic considerations. Clinical Pharmacokinetics 2002;41(2):115-35.

[67] de Wildt SN, van Schaik RH, Soldin OP, Soldin SJ, Brojeni PY, van der Heiden IP, Parshuram C, Nulman I, Koren G. The interactions of age, genetics, and disease severity on tacrolimus dosing requirements after pediatric kidney and liver transplantation. European Journal of Clinical Pharmacology 2011;67(12):1231-41.

[68] Cooney GF, Habucky K, Hoppu K. Cyclosporin pharmacokinetics in paediatric transplant recipients. Clinical Pharmacokinetics 1997;32(6):481-95.

[69] Jacqz-Aigrain E, Montes C, Brun P, Loirat C. Cyclosporine pharmacokinetics in nephrotic and kidney-transplanted children. European Journal of Clinical Pharmacology 1994;47(1):61-5.

[70] Staatz CE, Tett SE. Clinical pharmacokinetics and pharmacodynamics of tacrolimus in solid organ transplantation. Clinical Pharmacokinetics 2004;43(10):623-53.

[71] Fitzsimmons WE, Bekersky I, Dressler D, Raye K, Hodosh E, Mekki Q. Demographic considerations in tacrolimus pharmacokinetics. Transplantation Proceedings 1998;30(4): 1359-64.

[72] Mancinelli LM, Frassetto L, Floren LC, Dressler D, Carrier S, Bekersky I, Benet LZ, Christians U. The pharmacokinetics and metabolic disposition of tacrolimus: a comparison across ethnic groups. Clinical Pharmacology and Therapeutics 2001;69(1): 24-31.

[73] Ochiai T, Fukao K, Takahashi K, Endo T, Oshima S, Uchida K, Yokoyama I, Ishibashi M, Takahara S, Iwasaki Y. Phase III study of FK 506 in kidney transplantation. Japanese FK 506 Study Group. Transplantation Proceedings 1995;27(1):829-33.

[74] Citterio F. Evolution of the therapeutic drug monitoring of cyclosporine. Transplantation Proceedings 2004;36(2 Suppl):420S-425S.

[75] Trevillian P. Therapeutic drug monitoring. Nephrology 2007; 12, S57–S65.

[76] Kasiske BL, Heim-Duthoy K, Rao KV, Awni WM. The relationship between cyclosporin pharmacokinetic parameters and subsequent acute rejection in renal transplant recipients. Transplantation 1988;46: 716–22.

[77] Johnston A., Holt DW. Cyclosporine. In: Burton ME., Shaw LM., Schentag JJ., Evans WE. (ed) Applied Pharmacokinetics and Pharmacodynamics. Principles of Therapeutic Drug Monitoring. USA: Williams and Wilkins; 2006. p512-528.

[78] Dumont RJ, Ensom MH. Methods for clinical monitoring of cyclosporin in transplant patients. Clinical Pharmacokinetics 2000;38(5):427-47.

[79] Bauer LA. Applied Clinical Pharmacokinetics. USA: McGraw-Hill; 2001.

[80] Lindholm A, Kahan BD. Influence of cyclosporine pharmacokinetics, trough concentrations, and AUC monitoring on outcome after kidney transplantation. Clinical Pharmacology and Therapeutics 1993;54:205-18.

[81] Kahan BD, Welsh M, Schoenberg L, Rutzky LP, Katz SM, Urbauer DL, Van Buren CT. Variable oral absorption of cyclosporine. A biopharmaceutical risk factor for chronic renal allograft rejection. Transplantation 1996; 62:599-606.

[82] Levy GA. C2 monitoring strategy for optimizing cyclosporin immunosuppression from the Neoral formulation. BioDrugs 2001;15(5):279-90.

[83] David-Neto E, Araujo LP, Feres Alves C, Sumita N, Romano P, Yagyu EM, Nahas WC, Ianhez LE. A strategy to calculate cyclosporin A area under the time-concentration curve in pediatric renal transplantation. Pediatric Transplantation 2002;6(4):313-18.

[84] Weber LT, Armstrong VW, Shipkova M, Feneberg R, Wiesel M, Mehls O, Zimmerhackl LB, Oellerich M, Tönshoff B; Members of the German Study Group on Pediatric Renal Transplantion. Cyclosporin A absorption profiles in pediatric renal transplant recipients predict the risk of acute rejection. Therapeutic Drug Monitoring 2004;26(4):415-24.

[85] Mahalati K, Belitsky P, West K, Kiberd B, Fraser A, Sketris I, Macdonald AS, McAlister V, Lawen J. Approaching the therapeutic window for cyclosporine in kidney transplantation: a prospective study. Journal of the American Society of Nephrology 2001;12(4):828-33.

[86] Dunn CJ, Wagstaff AJ, Perry CM, Plosker GL, Goa KL. Cyclosporin: an updated review of the pharmacokinetic properties, clinical efficacy and tolerability of a microemulsion based formulation (neoral)1 in organ transplantation. Drugs 2001;61(13): 1957-2016.

[87] Keown PA. New concepts in cyclosporine monitoring. Current Opinion in Nephrology and Hypertension. 2002;11(6):619-26.

[88] Belitsky P, Dunn S, Johnston A, Levy G. Impact of absorption profiling on efficacy and safety of cyclosporin therapy in transplant recipients. Clinical Pharmacokinetics 2000;39(2):117-25.

[89] Grevel J, Post BK, Kahan BD. Michaelis-Menten kinetics determine cyclosporine steady-state concentrations: a population analysis in kidney transplant patients. Clinical Pharmacology and Therapeutics 1993;53(6):651-60. ABSTRACT

[90] Sheiner LB, Beal S, Rosenberg B, et al. Forecasting individual pharmacokinetics. Clinical Pharmacology & Therapeutics 1979;26:294-305.

[91] Jusko WJ, Thomson AW, Fung J, McMaster P, Wong SH, Zylber-Katz E, Christians U, Winkler M, Fitzsimmons WE, Lieberman R. Consensus document: therapeutic monitoring of tacrolimus (FK-506). Therapeutic Drug Monitoring 1995;17(6):606–614.

[92]   Staatz C, Taylor P, Tett S. Low tacrolimus concentrations and increased risk of early acute rejection in adult renal transplantation. Nephrology Dialysis and Transplantation 2001;16(9):1905-9.

[93]   Cattaneo D, Perico N, Remuzzi G. From pharmacokinetics to pharmacogenomics: a new approach to tailor immunosuppressive therapy. American Journal of Transplantation 2004;4(3):299-310.

[94]   Kapturczak MH, Meier-Kriesche HU, Kaplan B. Pharmacology of calcineurin antagonists. Transplantation Proceedings 2004;36(2 Suppl):25S-32S.

[95]   Scott LJ, McKeage K, Keam SJ, Plosker GL. Tacrolimus: a further update of its use in the management of organ transplantation. Drugs 2003;63(12):1247-97.

[96]   Jusko WJ, Kobayashi M. Therapeutic monitoring of tacrolimus (FK 506). Therapeutic Drug Monitoring 1993;15(4):349.

[97]   Shaw LM, Holt DW, Keown P, Venkataramanan R, Yatscoff RW. Current opinions on therapeutic drug monitoring of immunosuppressive drugs. Clinical Therapeutics 1999;21(10):1632-52.

[98]   Christians U., Pokaiyavanichkul T., Chan l. Tacrolimus. In: Applied Pharmacokinetics and Pharmacodynamics: Principles of Therapeutic Drug Monitoring, 4th Ed., edited by Burton ME, Shaw LM, Schentag JJ, Evans WE, Philadelphia, Lippincott Williams & Wilkins, 2006, pp 563–594.

[99]   Bullingham RES, Nicholls A, Hale M. Pharmacokinetics of mycophenolate mofetil (RS-61443): a short review. Transplantation Proceedings 1996;28:925-29.

[100]   Bullingham RE, Nicholls AJ, Kamm BR. Clinical Pharmacokinetics of Mycophenolate Mofetil. Clinical Pharmacokinetics 1998;34(6):429-455.

[101]   van Gelder T, Le Meur Y, Shaw LM, Oellerich M, DeNofrio D, Holt C, Holt DW, Kaplan B, Kuypers D, Meiser B, Toenshoff B, Mamelok RD. Therapeutic drug monitoring of mycophenolate mofetil in transplantation. Therapeutic Drug Monitoring 2006;28(2): 145-54.

[102]   Le Meur Y, Borrows R, Pescovitz MD, Budde K, Grinyo J, Bloom R, Gaston R, Walker RG, Kuypers D, van Gelder T, Kiberd B. Therapeutic drug monitoring of mycophenolates in kidney transplantation: report of The Transplantation Society consensus meeting. Transplantation Reviews 2011;25(2):58-64.

[103]   Nawrocki A., Korecka M., Solari S., Kang J., Shaw LM.: Mycophenolic acid. In: Applied Pharmacokinetics and Pharmacodynamics: Principles of Therapeutic Drug Monitoring, 4th Ed., edited by Burton ME, Shaw LM, Schentag JJ, Evans WE, Philadelphia, Lippincott Williams & Wilkins, 2006, pp 563–594.

[104]   Shaw LM, Figurski M, Milone MC, Trofe J, Bloom RD. Therapeutic drug monitoring of mycophenolic acid. Clinical Journal of the American Society of Nephrology 2007;2(5): 1062-72.

[105] Filler G, Mai I. Limited sampling strategy for mycophenolic acid area under the curve. Therapeutic Drug Monitoring 2000;22(2):169-73.

[106] Yeung S, Tong KL, Tsang WK, Tang HL, Fung KS, Chan HW, Chan AY, Chan L. Determination of mycophenolate area under the curve by limited sampling strategy. Transplantation Proceedings 2001;33(1-2):1052-3.

[107] Musuamba FT, Rousseau A, Bosmans JL, Senessael JJ, Cumps J, Marquet P, Wallemacq P, Verbeeck RK. Limited sampling models and Bayesian estimation for mycophenolic acid area under the curve prediction in stable renal transplant patients co-medicated with ciclosporin or sirolimus. Clinical Pharmacokinetics 2009;48(11):745-58.

[108] Pawinski T, Hale M, Korecka M, Fitzsimmons WE, Shaw LM. Limited sampling strategy for the estimation of mycophenolic acid area under the curve in adult renal transplant patients treated with concomitant tacrolimus. Clinical Chemistry 2002;48(9): 1497-504.

[109] Vasquez EM. Sirolimus: a new agent for prevention of renal allograft rejection. American Journal of Health System Pharmacy 2000; 57(7):437-48.

[110] Stenton SB, Partovi N, Ensom MH. Sirolimus: the evidence for clinical pharmacokinetic monitoring. Clinical Pharmacokinetics 2005;44(8):769-86.

[111] Ingle GR, Sievers TM, Holt CD. Sirolimus: continuing the evolution of transplant immunosuppression. Annals of Pharmacotherapy 2000;34:1044-55.

[112] Mahalati K, Kahan BD. Clinical Pharmacokinetics of Sirolimus. Clinical Pharmacokinetics 2001;40(8):573-585.

[113] Groth CG, Bäckman L, Morales JM, Calne R, Kreis H, Lang P, Touraine JL, Claesson K, Campistol JM, Durand D, Wramner L, Brattström C, Charpentier B. Sirolimus (rapamycin)-based therapy in human renal transplantation: similar efficacy and different toxicity compared with cyclosporine. Sirolimus European Renal Transplant Study Group. Transplantation 1999;67(7):1036-42.

[114] Hong JC, Kahan BD. Use of anti-CD25 monoclonal antibody in combination with rapamycin to eliminate cyclosporine treatment during the induction phase of immunosuppression. Transplantation 1999;68:701-4.

[115] Hong JC, Kahan BD. A calcineurin-free strategy for induction immunosuppression for delayed graft function in cadaveric kidney transplantation. Transplantation Proceedings 2001;33:1271-2.

[116] McAlister VC, Gao Z, Peltekian K, Domingues J, Mahalati K, MacDonald AS. Sirolimus-tacrolimus combination immunosuppression. Lancet 2000;355(9201):376-7.

[117] Zimmerman JJ, Kahan BD. Pharmacokinetics of sirolimus in stable renal transplant patients after multiple oral dose administration. Journal of Clinical Pharmacology 1997;37(5):405-15.

[118] Yatscoff RW, LeGatt DF, Kneteman NM. Therapeutic monitoring of rapamycin: a new immunosuppressive drug. Therapeutic Drug Monitoring 1993;15(6):478-82.

[119] Kirchner GI, Meier-Wiedenbach I, Manns MP. Clinical pharmacokinetics of everolimus. Clinical Pharmacokinetics. 2004;43(2):83-95.

[120] Kovarik JM, Kaplan B, Silva HT, Kahan BD, Dantal J, McMahon L, Berthier S, Hsu CH, Rordorf C. Pharmacokinetics of an everolimus-cyclosporine immunosuppressive regimen over the first 6 months after kidney transplantation. American Journal of Transplantation 2003;3(5):606-13.

[121] Budde K, Neumayer HH, Lehne G, Winkler M, Hauser IA, Lison A, Fritsche L, Soulillou JP, Fauchald P, Dantal J; RADW 102 Renal Transplant Study Group Tolerability and steady-state pharmacokinetics of everolimus in maintenance renal transplant patients. Nephrology Dialysis Transplantation 2004;19(10):2606-14.

[122] Helio Tedesco-Silva Jr, Claudia Rosso Felipe, Tainá Veras de Sandes, Freitas, Marina Pontello Cristeli, Carolina Araújo Rodrigues, José Osmar Medina Pestana. Impact of everolimus: update on immunosuppressive therapy strategies and patient outcomes after renal transplantation. Transplant Research and Risk Management 2011;3:9-29.

[123] Kovarik JM, Tedesco H, Pascual J, Civati G, Bizot MN, Geissler J, Schmidli H. Everolimus therapeutic concentration range defined from a prospective trial with reduced-exposure cyclosporine in de novo kidney transplantation. Therapeutic Drug Monitoring 2004;26(5):499-505.

[124] Mabasa VH, Ensom MH. The role of therapeutic monitoring of everolimus in solid organ transplantation. Therapeutic Drug Monitoring 2005;27(5):666-76.

[125] Shapiro R, Young JB, Milford EL, Trotter JF, Bustami RT, Leichtman AB. Immunosuppression: evolution in practice and trends, 1993-2003. American Journal of Transplantation 2005;5(4 Pt 2):874-86.

[126] Metalidis C, Kuypers DR. Emerging immunosuppressive drugs in kidney transplantation. Current Clinical Pharmacology 2011;6(2):130-6.

[127] Cooper JE, Wiseman AC. Novel immunosuppressive agents in kidney transplantation. Clinical Nephrology. 2010;73(5):333-43.

[128] Webber A, Hirose R, Vincenti F. Novel strategies in immunosuppression: issues in perspective. Transplantation 2011;91(10):1057-64.

[129] Kovarik JM, Steiger JU, Grinyo JM, Rostaing L, Arns W, Dantal J, Proot P, Budde K; Sotrastaurin Renal Transplant Study Group. Pharmacokinetics of sotrastaurin combined with tacrolimus or mycophenolic acid in de novo kidney transplant recipients. Transplantation 2011;91(3):317-22.

[130] Vincenti F, Charpentier B, Vanrenterghem Y, Rostaing L, Bresnahan B, Darji P, Massari P, Mondragon-Ramirez GA, Agarwal M, Di Russo G, Lin CS, Garg P, Larsen CP. A phase III study of belatacept-based immunosuppression regimens versus cyclosporine in renal transplant recipients (BENEFIT study). American Journal of Transplantation 2010;10(3):535-46.

Permissions

The contributors of this book come from diverse backgrounds, making this book a truly international effort. This book will bring forth new frontiers with its revolutionizing research information and detailed analysis of the nascent developments around the world.

We would like to thank Dr. med. Thomas Rath, for lending his expertise to make the book truly unique. He has played a crucial role in the development of this book. Without his invaluable contribution this book wouldn't have been possible. He has made vital efforts to compile up to date information on the varied aspects of this subject to make this book a valuable addition to the collection of many professionals and students.

This book was conceptualized with the vision of imparting up-to-date information and advanced data in this field. To ensure the same, a matchless editorial board was set up. Every individual on the board went through rigorous rounds of assessment to prove their worth. After which they invested a large part of their time researching and compiling the most relevant data for our readers. Conferences and sessions were held from time to time between the editorial board and the contributing authors to present the data in the most comprehensible form. The editorial team has worked tirelessly to provide valuable and valid information to help people across the globe.

Every chapter published in this book has been scrutinized by our experts. Their significance has been extensively debated. The topics covered herein carry significant findings which will fuel the growth of the discipline. They may even be implemented as practical applications or may be referred to as a beginning point for another development. Chapters in this book were first published by InTech; hereby published with permission under the Creative Commons Attribution License or equivalent.

The editorial board has been involved in producing this book since its inception. They have spent rigorous hours researching and exploring the diverse topics which have resulted in the successful publishing of this book. They have passed on their knowledge of decades through this book. To expedite this challenging task, the publisher supported the team at every step. A small team of assistant editors was also appointed to further simplify the editing procedure and attain best results for the readers.

Our editorial team has been hand-picked from every corner of the world. Their multi-ethnicity adds dynamic inputs to the discussions which result in innovative outcomes. These outcomes are then further discussed with the researchers and contributors who give their valuable feedback and opinion regarding the same. The feedback is then collaborated with the researches and they are edited in a comprehensive manner to aid the understanding of the subject.

Apart from the editorial board, the designing team has also invested a significant amount of their time in understanding the subject and creating the most relevant covers. They scrutinized every image to scout for the most suitable representation of the subject and create an appropriate cover for the book.

The publishing team has been involved in this book since its early stages. They were actively engaged in every process, be it collecting the data, connecting with the contributors or procuring relevant information. The team has been an ardent support to the editorial, designing and production team. Their endless efforts to recruit the best for this project, has resulted in the accomplishment of this book. They are a veteran in the field of academics and their pool of knowledge is as vast as their experience in printing. Their expertise and guidance has proved useful at every step. Their uncompromising quality standards have made this book an exceptional effort. Their encouragement from time to time has been an inspiration for everyone.

The publisher and the editorial board hope that this book will prove to be a valuable piece of knowledge for researchers, students, practitioners and scholars across the globe.

List of Contributors

Farzad Kakaei
Tabriz University of Medical Sciences, Tabriz, Iran

Saman Nikeghbalian and Seyed Ali Malekhosseini
Shiraz University of Medical Sciences, Shiraz, Iran

Katrien De Vusser and Maarten Naesens
Department of Nephrology and Renal Transplantation, University Hospitals Leuven, Leuven, Belgium

Lucan Mihai, Lucan Valerian Ciprian and Iacob Gheorghiță
Clinical Institute of Urology and Renal Transplantation, Cluj-Napoca, Romania

M. Ghanta, J. Dreier, R. Jacob and I. Lee
Section of Nephrology, Temple University School of Medicine, Philadelphia, PA, USA

A.A. Amir
Consultant Nephrologist, Dhahran Health Center, Saudi Aramco Medical Services Organization, Dhahran, Saudi Arabia

R.A. Amir
Dammam University, Dhahran, Saudi Arabia

S.S. Sheikh
Chief, Pathology and Laboratory Services, Dhahran Health Center, Saudi Aramco Medical Services Organization, Dhahran, Saudi Arabia

Thomas Rath and Stephan Ziefle
Department of Nephrology and Transplantation Medicine, Westpfalz-Klinikum GmbH, Kaiserslautern, Germany

Jean-Paul Squifflet
Department of Abdominal Surgery and Transplantation, University of Liege, Belgium

Rubina Naqvi
Nephrology Sindh Institute of Urology and Transplantation (SIUT), Karachi, Pakistan

María José Herrero and Virginia Bosó
Unidad de Farmacogenética, Instituto Investigación Sanitaria La Fe, Servicio de Farmacia, Hospital Universitario y Politécnico La Fe, Valencia, Spain

Luis Rojas
Unidad de Farmacogenética, Instituto Investigación Sanitaria La Fe, Servicio de Farmacia, Hospital Universitario y Politécnico La Fe, Valencia, Spain
Hospital clínico de la Pontificia Universidad Católica de Chile, Dpto. Medicina Interna, y Centro de Investigaciones Clínicas, Chile

Sergio Bea, Jaime Sánchez Plumed and Julio Hernández
Servicio Nefrología, Hospital Universitario y Politécnico La Fe, Valencia, Spain

Jose Luis Poveda
Servicio de Farmacia, Hospital Universitario y Politécnico La Fe, Valencia, Spain

Salvador F. Aliño
Unidad Farmacología Clínica, Hospital Universitario y Politécnico La Fe, Dpto. Farmacología, Fac. Medicina, Universidad de Valencia, Valencia, Spain

Ana Luisa Robles Piedras, Minarda De la O Arciniega and Josefina Reynoso Vázquez
Academic Area of Pharmacy, Institute of Health Sciences, Autonomous University of Hidalgo State, Mexico

Printed in the USA
CPSIA information can be obtained
at www.ICGtesting.com
JSHW011408221024
72173JS00003B/456

9 781632 410245